AURAL HABILITATION:

The Foundations of Verbal Learning in Hearing-Impaired Children

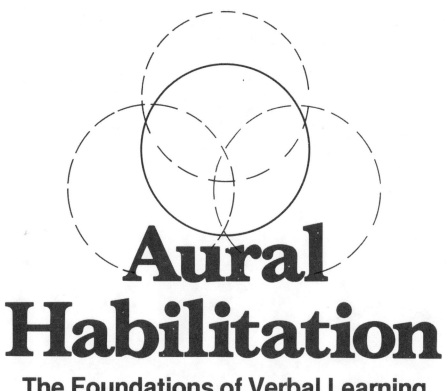

Aural Habilitation

The Foundations of Verbal Learning in Hearing-Impaired Children

Daniel Ling and Agnes H. Ling

The Alexander Graham Bell Association for the Deaf
3417 Volta Place, N.W., Washington, D.C. 20007, U.S.A.
Library of Congress Catalogue Card Number 78-56077
ISBN 0-88200-121-3

Preface

This book is intended as a text for students of audiology, speech pathology, or special education. It is also written for teachers and clinicians, educational administrators, and parents. It describes the form and content of work that can lead to effective speech communication skills among hearing-impaired children.

To optimize readability we have, so far as possible, omitted references from the text. We have included annotated bibliographies at the end of each chapter for those who wish to study any topic in greater detail. To avoid certain complexities we refer to teachers or clinicians as "she" and the child as "he," and apologize to readers who are annoyed by such a sexist convention. We wish to thank our sons Philip and Alister for their various contributions to this text, Carole Shevloff for typing it, Max Steibel and Wim Van Eyk of the Instructional Communications Center of McGill University for the illustrations, and Bettie Loux Donley for her work as editor, designer, and producer. We are also grateful to our students and to our colleagues at McGill University for their constant encouragement and support.

The publication of this book was made possible through a grant from the Western Electric Fund of New York.

International Phonetic Alphabet Symbols
Representing Speech Sounds and Modifiers

Consonants

Symbol	Key Word
[p]	*p*ea
[b]	*b*ee
[t]	*t*ea
[d]	*d*o
[k]	*k*ey
[g]	*g*o
[m]	*m*y
[n]	*n*o
[ŋ]	Li*ng*
[h]	*h*op
[f]	*f*ee
[v]	*v*ery
[θ]	*th*in
[ð]	*th*at
[s]	*s*o
[z]	*z*oo
[ʃ]	*sh*e
[ʒ]	ca*s*ual
[tʃ]	*ch*eap
[dʒ]	*j*eep
[ʍ]	*wh*ey
[w]	*w*e
[j]	*y*ou
[r]	*r*ed
[l]	*l*ook

Vowels

Symbol	Key Word
[u]	wh*o*
[ʊ]	w*ou*ld
[o]	kn*o*w
[ɔ]	m*o*re
[ɑ]	*o*f
[a]	*a*rt
[ʌ]	m*u*st
[ɝ]	l*ea*rn
[ə]	*a*gain
[ɚ]	moth*er*
[æ]	*a*nd
[ɛ]	th*e*n
[e]	ta*ke*
[ɪ]	h*i*s
[i]	*ea*se

Diphthongs

Symbol	Key Word
[aɪ]	p*ie*
[aʊ]	c*ow*
[ɔɪ]	t*oy*
[eɪ]	pl*ay*
[ɪɚ]	h*ere*

Modifiers

[ʰ]	aspirated
[ₒ]	voiceless
[⁻]	unreleased
[.]	syllabic consonant

Table of Contents

List of Figures

List of Tables

*This book is dedicated to those
who truly wish hearing-impaired children
to be able to speak for themselves.*

1. Introduction

Most hearing-impaired children can learn to speak and understand spoken language if they are given adequate opportunity to do so. Adequate opportunity can be provided only if those concerned with a child's care —parents, teachers, clinicians, and administrators —are aware of, and exploit, the conditions that contribute to verbal learning. The purpose of this text is to discuss knowledge and skills relating to verbal learning and to describe how they can be employed in the aural habilitation of hearing-impaired children. It is written for parents, teacher/clinicians, and administrators who are currently involved with hearing-impaired children, and is intended to provide introductory material for students in the fields of speech pathology, audiology, psychology, and education.

Scope of the Text

We begin our treatment of verbal learning with a brief description of the various aspects of communication (Chapter 2). We discuss verbal and nonverbal communication, the distinction between speech and language, and the social implications of being able to speak and understand speech. We also describe how different degrees of hearing loss can affect the ability of adults to communicate, and how hearing impairment may hinder the development of verbal learning in children.

The normal development of spoken language is described in Chapter 3. Knowledge of this process helps the parent and

1

teacher/clinician to follow a natural path of treatment when habilitation is begun in the first year or so of life. It further helps to devise strategies to foster verbal skills in older children—those whose linguistic development has been retarded by delay in the diagnosis and treatment of hearing impairment. Older children cannot simply recapitulate the process of language development observed in younger children, as this would not accord with their greater social and cognitive maturity. But neither can they be taught fluent verbal skills through reference to rules and notions imposed upon them. Hearing-impaired children, like their normal-hearing counterparts, must derive the rules which govern the meaningful use of spoken language for themselves, through abundant experience of communicative speech. Our focus upon the normal process of language development is deliberate, for hearing impairment does not change the basic nature of a child's central nervous system and how it best deals with verbal material.

The central nervous system of a hearing-impaired child, unless severe brain damage is also involved, is tuned by nature to process spoken language patterns. The problem faced in aural habilitation is, essentially, how best to supply the child's central nervous system with verbal patterns that are sufficiently clear and sufficiently frequent to activate this processing capability and to develop it. In short, the task is to ensure that hearing impairment does not prevent verbal stimuli from reaching the child's central nervous system through one sense modality or another. The various ways in which the senses can be engaged in this task are discussed in later chapters.

Of course, audition is the most appropriate sense modality for speech reception. Even when hearing is impaired, its role should, if possible, be given primary emphasis. If the utmost use is to be made of residual hearing, those concerned with hearing-impaired children must have at least a basic knowledge of the sound patterns of speech and language, how they are classified, how they are perceived, and how they differ acoustically. We treat these matters in Chapter 4. Inevitably, the treatment is somewhat technical, but not overwhelmingly so. Since the acoustic patterns of speech are the raw material of verbal interchange, the information here presented is essential to understanding the problems posed by hearing impairment.

Hearing impairment, as we imply above, is not an all-or-none affair. Like visual impairment, it can be present as a mild deficit which causes no significant handicap, as a total loss of sensory function, or as a partial loss of acuity lying somewhere between these two extremes. Total deafness is extremely rare, hence most children can hear at least some speech patterns if sound is adequately amplified for them. Hearing impairment may stem from a variety of causes, be present at birth, or occur at any subsequent time. Some types of hearing impairment, those affecting the outer or middle ear, may be amenable to medical or surgical treatment and hence temporary in nature. Others, those affecting the inner ear (the cochlea) or the auditory nerve, can not be cured by any known procedure. In this text we do not discuss causation or medical/surgical treatment. Our concern is with the habilitation of those children (about one in a thousand born in most populations) whose hearing impairment is permanent and shown by audiologic assessment to be sufficiently severe as to hinder or prevent verbal learning if it is left untreated. In Chapter 5 we describe the behavioral and instrumental tests that are commonly employed in audiologic assessment and how they are used as a basis for planning treatment.

Fundamental to aural habilitation is the selection, fitting, and use of hearing aids. In Chapter 6, we stress that there is no such thing as a hearing aid that will suit all children, and that amplification needs will depend upon the nature and extent of each individual's hearing impairment. We describe how amplification needs can be estimated, what factors govern the selection of appropriate instruments, and how our Five-Sound Test and other measures of hearing can be used to determine the validity of a hearing aid selection procedure. We discuss monaural and binaural fittings and present our rationale for recommending two aids in preference to one.

We continue our description and discussion of hearing aids in Chapter 7, which is devoted to the use of residual audition. Our treatment of this aspect derives from our view that, once selected and fitted, hearing aids should be regarded as an integral part of the child's auditory system, which begins at the microphone of each instrument and ends at the brain. We emphasize the need for special-purpose hearing aids (hard-wire, loop, and radio systems) in certain circumstances, in order to ensure optimal detection of the speech signal and the comprehension and use of the spoken word. We explain why we consider auditory discrimination and identification exercises to have limited value. We do not entirely reject the notion of "auditory training" but suggest that, given appropriate hearing aids, auditory experience of spoken language in meaningful, real-life situations provides a superior basis for developing full use of a child's residual hearing.

The more severely a child's hearing is impaired, the greater must be the emphasis on speech reception through alternative sense modalities. In Chapter 8, we describe how vision may be employed to serve as a supplement or as an alternative to the use of residual audition, and how touch can assist in the development of speech. We stress the weaknesses of speechreading and suggest procedures by which one can augment the limited and ambiguous information a child can obtain from speechread patterns.

Ability to produce the sound patterns of a language is, of course, essential if the child is to express himself fluently through speech communication. Such ability also assists a child in the speech reception task, in that the child who is able to speak can use his knowledge of phonology as a matrix against which to interpret incoming information and as a means of rehearsing and storing language patterns in short- and long-term memory. We describe the process of speech acquisition (Chapter 9) as one which involves numerous sequential stages, each providing the prerequisite skills for the development of subsequent stages. Although we discuss speech evaluation in some detail and suggest a simplified procedure for the assessment of phonologic speech skills, our primary focus is upon the integration of speech teaching, language learning, and the use of residual audition. We indicate how auditory training can, if necessary, be systematically undertaken in the context of both phonetic and phonologic speech teaching. We also present and describe a new model for evoking and generalizing speech target behaviors. This model, based on an analysis of videotapes of speech work undertaken by a variety of teacher/clinicians, provides a rationale for the selection of the most appropriate sense modality (modalities) in the speech teaching task. A further concern in this chapter is with the transfer of phonetic level skills into phonologic speech, and we suggest strategies by which such transfer can be achieved.

In Chapter 10, we describe how the type of interaction that normally takes place between parent and child in the first year of life can be fostered in hearing-impaired infants and their parents. Here we seek to indicate how the information provided in previous chapters can be applied. We indicate the rationale for early diagnosis and habilitation and suggest the type of counseling that should accompany audiologic assessment and hearing aid fitting. We outline the strategies that assist the child in developing basic listening and motor speech skills and their use in vocal and verbal communication.

Language development has long been recognized as the most basic need of hearing-impaired children, and the most important task of their teachers. Over time, various methods for teaching language skills have been put forward. Most have involved the presentation and assessment of language through vision—particularly the written form—and most have required formal instruction based upon grammatical analysis. Relatively few children have achieved normal linguistic skills through such instruction. In Chapter 11, we suggest that hearing-impaired children should not be taught through a grammatical approach, but should be helped to derive the rules which underlie the meaningful use of the spoken word through abundant experience in speech communication. We do not suggest that the process of verbal learning should be haphazard. Rather, we emphasize how meaning can be conveyed through reference to the child's interests and ongoing activities so that the speaker's intent becomes apparent to him. We suggest that those in contact with the child can encourage verbal comprehension and, as it develops, systematically increase the complexity and variety of language forms while decreasing the child's reliance on nonverbal cues. The problems relating to the assessment of emerging linguistic skills are also discussed.

Hearing children learn how to read and write after they have learned to talk. Written language, for them, is learned in relation to the sound patterns they hear and produce. They learn the written form as one which corresponds closely to (and represents) their speech. In Chapter 12 we suggest that most hearing-impaired children can, and should, follow the normal sequence of events and be introduced to reading and writing only when they have a substantial background of spoken language. Few children are developmentally ready to read and write before 5 or 6 years of age, by which time basic spoken language skills can usually be established if habilitation is begun in the first year or so of life. Of course, reading and writing can be forced upon younger children, but acquisition of these skills will be less rapid than if they are left for a year or two. We recognize that language, speech, reading, and writing skills can be taught together, but consider that such practice imposes a burden that is unnecessarily great, one that is likely to discourage the development of fluency and the enrichment of vocabulary, language, thought, and knowledge that comes through reading for pleasure.

In Chapter 13 we describe the various forms of special education provision that exist for hearing-impaired children and discuss the opportunities for verbal learning that each can provide. We indicate what questions parents and teacher/clinicians should have in mind when seeking to determine whether a special education program can meet the individual needs of a given child. Finally, in Chapter 14, we analyze the range of knowledge and skills that is required of teacher/clinicians if they are to work effectively in the field of aural habilitation. We conclude that there are currently few professionals who can truthfully claim to possess the full range of competencies that are essential. We hope that our analysis will stimulate the creation of improved training programs, some geared to prepare more highly qualified teacher/clinicians and others designed to upgrade the skills of those who are currently engaged in the field. Without such programs, many hearing-impaired children will not achieve their potential for verbal learning.

Exclusions From the Text

Since this work is concerned with the foundations of spoken language development, we make but passing reference to the use of manual communication (sign language and/or fingerspelling). To debate the relative merits of different philosophies would simply detract from our purpose, which is to present introductory material on aspects of knowledge that are directly and fundamentally related to the development of verbal skills. Our bias is both widely known and evident from the contents of this book. We believe that every child whose parents wish it should be given optimal opportunity to learn spoken language. We believe that, initially at least, such opportunity is best provided by the abundant use of spoken language without signs or fingerspelling. We hope that those who do not share our views will nevertheless find the material presented in this text to be of value, since the need for spoken language teaching is generally accepted regardless of educational philosophy.

We recognize that a small proportion of children cannot acquire fluent spoken language skills. Discussion of their treatment is not attempted in this text. We stress, however, that identification of such children can only be made on the basis of evaluations carried out in the course of ongoing treatment. Degree of hearing impairment, intelligence, parental concern and ability, and additional handicaps as assessed on initial diagnoisis cannot reliably indicate whether a child will be able to communicate verbally. Totally deaf children given skilled attention *can* learn to speak. Indeed, we know many oral deaf adults whose speech, acquired without benefit of hearing, is so intelligible that they are capable of giving lectures to large audiences. Intelligence, except in the very severely mentally retarded, is known to have little relationship with ability to acquire speech. In any case, the measurement of intelligence in babies, normal-hearing and hearing-impaired, is prone to considerable error. Parental concern and ability are also hard to quantify, particularly prior to the initiation of training; at this point parents are having to deal with their feelings of guilt, grief, anxiety, and bewilderment. How well parents can adjust and contribute to the development of their child's spoken language largely depends on the quality of counseling they receive. Whether parents are motivated to acquire the knowledge and skills they need in order to cope efficiently with their hearing-impaired child can be as much a measure of the teacher/clinician's competence as of parental capacity. Certain handicaps in addition to hearing impairment do not prevent spoken language development, although they may slow the rate of acquisition. For example, we worked with a severely hearing-impaired child who was also blind in one eye and partially sighted in the other and so retarded in motor development that she could not sit up unsupported until 15 months of age. This child, now 12 years old, has received all of her education in regular schools, is at grade level in mathematics, one year below grade level in reading, but bilingual in French and English.

The main thrust of this text is toward habilitation rather than rehabilitation—toward the development rather than the remediation of verbal skills. To be sure, many of the topics treated are relevant to such remedial work with older children, but our main concern in this text is principally with the younger child. Our rationale is that if severe spoken language deficits are to be prevented, then much more attention has to be given to the treatment of hearing impairment during infancy and early childhood. Of course the remedial treatment of the older child is important and, at present, more extensive than preventative work with children aged 0-6 years. In the absence of early habilitation, however, remedial work is analogous to treating an overflowing bath by pulling out the plug and not turning off the tap. There will be no abatement in the number of children requiring remedial work in later school life unless more adequate provision is made for children in their first few years of life. By limiting our discussion mainly to younger children we hope to encourage more extensive and effective early treatment; then hopefully, in the years ahead, fewer older children will have to face the problems that are currently experienced by those in school and at college. That there is a need to re-order priorities is evident. We can point to numerous young people who left special schools with unintelligible speech and impoverished language and are now learning to speak clearly and in acceptable English as a result of good remedial teaching. Why were these young adults not given the opportunity to develop spoken language skills as children? Speech communication skills permit access to society at large, and to restrict or deny opportunity to develop such skills from early infancy is to impose social and intellectual deprivation upon the child already handicapped by hearing impairment.

We have, as far as possible, excluded references. We decided that to do so would enhance the readability of the material which, in parts, is unavoidably complex. We have, instead, provided an annotated bibliography at the end of each chapter for those readers who wish to pursue specific topics in more depth. In these bibliographies we list a few reviews which themselves contain useful references, but have mainly suggested selected books that provide more comprehensive coverage and are readily accessible either commercially or through libraries. There are, of course, many journals which contain material relevant to this text. Of particular relevance is *The Volta Review*, the journal of the Alexander Graham Bell Association for the Deaf.

An Orientation

In addition to students, this book is intended for parents, teacher/clinicians, and administrators. The three groups may appear to have little in common. Yet, if the hearing-impaired child is to succeed in learning to use spoken language, it is essential that these groups function as a team, each understanding and having respect for the others' roles in the habilitation process. Indeed, the principle of such collaboration is embodied in U.S. Public Law 94–142. In the following paragraphs and throughout this text we present material that is fundamental to such understanding and, by interrelating information presented in different chapters, indicate how collaboration by those concerned can benefit the individual child. Although the habilitation process broadly follows a similar sequence for all children, we emphasize that the range of differences to be found among children is so large that optimal progress can only be assured through individual attention. One may have similar goals for a variety of children, but the strategies employed to reach these goals must be selected in the light of each child's needs.

Parents

This book is designed as much for parents as for the professionals who will help them to achieve the goals they desire for their children. Parents (or guardians) are the most important people in a hearing-impaired child's life.

1. *Parents are, with very few exceptions, the individuals who are most concerned about the development of the child.* Parents have the overall responsibility for their children. Although professionals may be concerned with how their contributions can help a child achieve particular skills that are essential to his overall development, they cannot give the child the amount of individual attention, love, and consistent long-term care that will enable the child to develop to his full human potential.

2. *Parents can do more than professionals to help the child develop verbal skills in early infancy.* The development of spoken language in infancy requires abundant verbal interaction between adult and child on a one-to-one basis. It also requires that what is said to the child relates to his interests and ongoing activities. Only the parents, who are available to the infant during all waking hours, can provide the wealth of meaningful spoken language experiences that is required to promote his comprehension and use of speech. Helping a hearing-impaired child to acquire native mastery of language is almost a full-time occupation for a parent over a three- to four-year period. It is during the first three to four years of life that conditions are optimal for language learning.

3. *Only parents can provide continuity of care.* No single profes-

sional is likely to be available to a child on a long-term basis. Doctors, teachers, and clinicians come and go. They move out of town or are required to work with other children. It is therefore in the best interests of the child for the parent to become well-informed so that continuity of care and effort is ensured at each stage of development.

4. *Early intervention is most effective when parents are involved.* Studies of early efforts to stimulate language growth in infants have shown that the results are best and most enduring when parents are directly involved and when the mother sees herself as being the most important contributor to the child's progress.

5. *The parents' role largely determines the future of a hearing-impaired child.* The evidence on this point is clear. Behind the successful oral deaf adults of earlier generations and the highly verbal hearing-impaired young adults of today, one can usually find dedicated parents. In most cases such parents have gone out of their way to seek out the best professional advice and apply it whole-heartedly They have enlisted the aid of professionals, but have never assigned them primary responsibility for their child's verbal development.

Given competent professional support and guidance soon after hearing impairment is suspected, most parents can help their children learn to talk. When guidance is inadequate, and when there is a long delay before referral and the onset of a guidance program, parents may well become convinced that they cannot handle the task. Of course, there are parents who are either unwilling or unable to become involved in a parent-infant program. Although it is necessary to respect their viewpoint, serious attempts should be made to ensure that parents are aware of the implications.

There are also children, what percentage we do not know, who for various reasons may be unable to develop spoken language, even with the most willing of parents and the most competent of professionals. A large number of such children have major handicaps in addition to hearing impairment. However, the presence of such additional problems should not automatically rule out the initial use of an auditory-oral approach. Whatever the extent of the child's problems and whatever training procedure is recommended, the hearing-impaired child is likely to develop optimally only if his parents realize their crucial role, and seek counsel, guidance, and support from professionals with proven skills.

This text is intended to indicate the variety of ways in which parents can help their children, and to describe the type and content of support and guidance that they can expect from professional workers. It is also intended to acquaint them with ways in which administrators can work toward the provision of comprehensive services, and how parents can be involved in the placement of their children in the most appropriate educational setting. Parents are entitled to participate in the development of individualized educational programs for their children. They should not hesitate to exercise this right.

Teacher/Clinicians

We consider the primary role of teacher/clinicians who deal with hearing-impaired children in their early years to be the support and guidance of the parents. Teacher/clinicians should ensure that the potential for the child's spoken language development in the home is enhanced through their efforts, and that this potential is exploited to promote the foundation of language before the child is admitted to a school-based program. Parent-oriented endeavor should precede but also accompany child-oriented work at later stages. Knowledge and skills that can be acquired by parents in the early stages can help them support the teacher/clinician when the child is ready to attend school.

Teacher/clinicians, both by training and by inclination, are too frequently tempted to work directly with the child rather than with his parents. There is a natural attraction to interacting directly with a young child, and considerable satisfaction to be gained from personally helping the child to achieve a particular target behavior. However, enduring effects on the child's spoken communication will be obtained only if the parents are able to reinforce and extend the child's range of behaviors through their own efforts—efforts that should persist throughout the child's life and enrich later out-of-school experience.

Teacher/clinicians often recommend early admission to a nursery or other placement in the belief that their specialist skills will allow them to achieve more than the parents. Caution should be exercised in this regard. Too early placement of a child in a school-based program should be as strongly avoided as undue delay in admission to a program for which he is developmentally prepared. Placement in a nursery class with hearing-impaired children who are unable to talk can drastically impede the progress of a child who has begun to communicate through speech. Such placement is of equally little benefit to a child who has not begun to talk, for it will provide but restricted exposure to normal patterns of speech and behavior. Early placement in a nursery may also result in the child repeating a year of pre-school with the result that he becomes bored with the activities and develops poor attitudes to learning. Teacher/clinicians' skills are best exercised directly with the child when they have first been used effectively with parents, and the foundations of verbal learning have been firmly established through a parent-infant program.

What are the tasks of a parent-oriented teacher/clinician? We believe that they should include the following ten activities:

1. *Helping parents accept the facts and implications of their child's problems as they become known.* This task involves providing parents with explanations of audiological and other diagnostic tests, discussing the results of these tests with them, and explaining how findings relate to the design of an individual plan for the habilitation of their child. Parents should neither be under-informed nor given so much detail that it cannot be absorbed. Tests and assessments undertaken in the course of parent-infant training should be similarly discussed. The informed parent is the greatest resource for both the child and the teacher/clinician (see Chapters 5 and 10).

2. *Helping parents acquire the confidence to cope with the child.* Parents need to have feedback on their effectiveness and reinforcement for their efforts if they are to acquire the confidence that is essential to their successful handling of the child. The most effective form of feedback and reinforcement is evident achievement. If the teacher/clinician sets well-defined short-term goals for the child, then parents can readily see for themselves when progress is being made. Description and demonstration of the strategies that will help the parents achieve success in realization of such goals, and confirmation that the child has achieved them, are therefore basic to parent guidance (see Chapters 9–12).

3. *Helping parents to acquire suitable hearing aids for the child and ensuring their optimal use.* Hearing aids are the most valuable tool available for aural habilitation. Every teacher/clinician working with young children should be familiar with selection and fitting procedures and should be able to explain them to the parents. Beyond that, they should help the parents accept the child's needs for amplification and teach the parent how to care for the hearing

aids, check their adequacy, and encourage the child to listen and learn through the use of residual hearing (see Chapters 6 and 7).

4. *Helping parents to establish eye-to-eye contact with their child in communication.* Eye-to-eye contact is an essential part of communication (see Chapters 2 and 10). To insist upon eye-to-eye contact is not to place emphasis on vision rather than hearing. Children with whom eye-to-eye contact is customary from early infancy are, however, ready to develop whatever speechreading skills they may require to supplement the input they receive through the use of residual audition (see Chapter 8).

5. *Helping parents to persist in stimulating the child's efforts to use voice and communicate through speech.* At every stage of development, the child should receive encouragement to use voice and speech. At the outset, parents can simply reinforce the child's vocalizations. As the child acquires more of the sound patterns of language, parents may be expected to help him rehearse particular vowels or syllables and motivate the child to use them consistently in conversation (see Chapters 9–11).

6. *Helping parents to develop skills of observation and listening.* Teacher/clinicians are enormously aided in their work if parents are able to report with accuracy the child's responses to sounds and his attempts at speech. Children are not always ready to perform, and problems do not necessarily become apparent during the child's visits to the parent-infant guidance center or during the teacher/clinician's visit to the child's home. Accurate observation and reporting on the part of parents may alert the teacher/clinician to the need for an adjustment to the child's hearing aids, lead her to suggest strategies for preventing unwanted behaviors, or help her to formulate methods of extending the use of speech patterns that will be of especial appeal to a particular child (see Chapter 10).

7. *Helping parents to create and exploit natural and informal situations in the child's everyday life that make language more readily meaningful to him.* Every home is governed by certain routines that not only develop a child's sense of security, but provide the repetition and situational structure that are essential for language learning. For example, young children may put on and take off clothes as many as six times a day. Parent-child conversations about such a simple activity can be used to introduce an enormous range of vocabulary and language structures. They would include words such as "off," "on," "hot," "cold," "wet," "dress," "coat," "shirt,"

"socks," and phrases like "too small," "too large," "I'm too hot," "It's dirty," "Take it off." Six occasions a day provide more than 2,000 opportunities for repetition and extensions of spoken language a year on a one-to-one basis. Other routines—such as toilet, bathing, meals, and preparation for bed—provide similar meaningful opportunities for the child to learn spoken language forms. Further routines can be created through play. Parents do not have to be rich or highly educated to provide their child with a wealth of language. Most, however, need to be shown how to make the most of situations that promote verbal learning in the context of everyday life. Such situations are far more meaningful and abundant than those most teacher/clinicians can supply in a program that limits opportunity for one-to-one interaction.

8. *Helping parents provide opportunities for the all-round integrated development of the child as a whole person and as an essential member of his family and society.* No man, woman, or child is an island. One's relationships with others are the predominant feature of human life. How well the parents help a hearing-impaired child to develop feelings of self-worth in the framework of the family will largely determine his future relationships with others. His parents must consider him as a child first, and a hearing-impaired child next. His needs and interests are primarily the same as those of normal-hearing children of the same age. Only if he is given every opportunity to participate in the activities enjoyed by normal-hearing children will his hearing impairment ever become a matter of secondary importance.

9. *Helping parents to achieve consistently firm but affectionate handling of the child.* There is a tendency for parents to be exceptionally lenient in their handling of a hearing-impaired child, to adopt more permissive standards than they would usually set for normal-hearing children. This tendency can result in behavioral disorders that have disastrous effects on the child's verbal learning. The limits set for acceptable behavior should conform to those which the parents would adopt with normal-hearing children. It is essential that limits, when set, should be consistently upheld.

10. *Helping parents to meet the needs of their hearing-impaired child without jeopardizing the well-being of the family as a whole.* Parents often need guidance in dealing with a hearing-impaired child in such a way that their attention is adequately shared and that harmony is maintained among all members of the family. The exten-

sive attention required by the hearing-impaired child may engender feelings of jealousy and even hate among others in the family group. Parents can often be helped, by a discussion of the problem, to devise ways to give the child the attention he needs and to reserve for others the time that they require. They may also explore the possibilities of receiving help from others, either relations, friends, members of their social group, or neighbors if the need arises. It is very easy for an overly conscientious mother to spend so much time coping with her hearing-impaired child and with her other children that she becomes jaded and depressed. It is not in anyone's interest that such a situation should be allowed to occur. Her well-being is essential and her concern should not be permitted to prevent her from obtaining adequate relaxation and recreation. The skilled teacher/clinician should therefore be aware of the needs of parents as well as those of the children.

Our emphasis upon the role of the teacher/clinician in parent-infant work does not imply a lack of concern with the application of her special skills in school-based programs. This is evident from the content of Chapters 9–13. But what is actually special in the needs of hearing-impaired children? Clearly it is their need to develop effective verbal skills. Given these skills, the barriers to communication and learning can be overcome.

Administrators

So many individual differences exist among children with hearing impairment that no single form of educational provision can possibly meet the variety of their needs. In this text we specify the conditions which lead to verbal learning—a factor which contributes to further individual differences. We indicate why provision should include programs for the habilitation of hearing-impaired children from early infancy, what qualifications personnel appointed for this work should have, and the nature of the work that they should undertake.

If a substantial proportion of hearing-impaired children is to be absorbed into mainstream educational settings in accordance with the spirit of U.S. Public Law 94–142, special help of the type described in this text must be afforded to a greater number of hearing-impaired children from early infancy. It is certainly within the power of most administrators to effect changes in provision that will lead to the placement of more hearing-impaired children in regular schools. Of course, we do not suggest that all hearing-impaired children can or should be so placed. Some children—those unable to benefit from regular school placement—would be less restricted in their opportunity for education if taught within special settings. Options must include placement within regular classes with the necessary support services to maintain such placement, special services to foster partial integration, and self-contained schools or classes for those who cannot benefit from full- or part-time placement in the mainstream of education.

It is rare for improvements in education to be associated with long-term reduction of expenditures. Yet analysis of the relative costs of various types of provision clearly demonstrates the financial advantages of placing emphasis on early and effective aural habilitation and the development of spoken language. Mainstreamed hearing-impaired children who require support services are considerably less expensive to educate than those in special self-contained schools or classes. Day school or day class provision costs much less than residential school placements. By implementing programs of early verbal training which can, if efficiently run, lead to the majority of hearing-impaired children being mainstreamed, administrators can enhance potential for the personal-social development of many, and effect substantial savings in so doing.

One of the goals of education is to prepare the child for adult life. Children currently being educated, and those who will shortly enter the school system, are destined to live most of their lives in the 21st century. In order to live happily and support themselves and their families in the years ahead, flexibility in the acquisition of skills that will allow them to adapt to technological advances will be required. Verbal communication—and the reading skills which derive from it —will continue to be the most important avenue of learning and adaptation. Hearing-impaired adults with effective speech skills currently enjoy better socioeconomic standing than those who cannot speak. Those who cannot speak require many more special services throughout their lives than those who can. Emphasis in education must therefore be placed upon early verbal learning.

The literature on hearing-impaired children indicates that optimal opportunities for the development of verbal learning and adequate preparation for placement in regular classes are provided when the following eight conditions are met:

1. *Early detection of hearing impairment.* Because relatively few children are identified as having hearing impairment in the first year of life, diagnosis and provision of services are generally delayed. Such delay can be prevented if those in administrative positions work with medical and paramedical personnel to promote public awareness of hearing impairment and to organize adequate referral systems.

2. *Early admission of hearing-impaired children to programs that offer continuity of assessment and treatment.* For children detected as hearing-impaired in the first year of life, admission to a parent-infant program should be immediate. We describe the assessment and habilitation procedures that can be employed in such a program and emphasize that assessment must be considered as part of ongoing training. A teacher/clinician with the appropriate skills can deal with at least 12 families, each on a one-to-one basis, through weekly guidance sessions. In the course of these sessions, she can continue the diagnostic process and guide parents in the habilitation of the child (see Chapters 5–12). For children detected up to age 3 or 4, parent-infant programs can usually offer more than immediate admission to a special class (see above). Even following admission to a special class, continued diagnosis and assessment of a child's needs for amplification (Chapters 6–7) and verbal training (Chapters 9–12) should proceed in parallel with his habilitation.

3. *Full-time use of appropriate amplification.* Hearing aids should be considered as educational rather than medical equipment, since their primary use is as a tool that enables a child to learn. Failure to provide hearing-impaired children with appropriate amplification not only impedes their progress, but wastes the time and skills of the teacher/clinician. At current prices, two hearing aids can be provided for less than $500. They can be expected to last for at least five years, and can be run for less than $100/year. Children who are not provided with appropriate amplification cannot be taught as effectively as those who have adequate hearing aids (see Chapters 6 and 7). The cost to an educational program if a child does not have appropriate hearing aids can be calculated as the sum of (a) a substantial proportion of the teacher/clinician's salary (time effectively lost) and (b) the expenses that will be incurred in providing the child with special educational treatment for an unnecessarily extensive period — perhaps the rest of the child's school life. The cost of appropriate

amplification is clearly the less. Failure to ensure that children are using suitable hearing aids all of their waking hours is an enormous weakness in current educational provision for hearing-impaired children.

4. *A highly competent teacher/clinician to work frequently, intensively, and individually with the child and his parents.* Teacher/clinicians who have all or even most of the competencies required for aural habilitation are rare. Indeed, the low standards of language and educational achievement that generally prevail among hearing-impaired children can be largely attributed to the widespread employment of inadequately trained personnel. Administrators can do much to remedy the situation through recognizing the need, and creating a demand, for teacher/clinicians who have fulfilled more than the currently accepted minimal training requirements—personnel whose training has been specifically for the work they are required to do. The range of knowledge and skills required by teacher/clinicians if they are to be maximally effective is discussed throughout this text and is the topic specifically treated in Chapter 14. Support for initial training of new personnel and the upgrading of those currently employed must be considered as priorities by those in administrative positions.

5. *Parents who collaborate in the child's treatment program.* The extent of parental collaboration required has already been discussed in preceding sections. As indicated throughout this text, we would like to promote ways of helping parents to act as the primary agents in aural habilitation—and in any case, consider them as essential members of the habilitation team. We fully support the opportunities provided for them to participate in the educational process under U.S. Public Law 94–142.

6. *Extensive exposure of the child to spoken language patterns that should be common to both home and school.* If a child is to learn English language patterns, then he must be adequately exposed to normal models, models which can be provided only by native or fluent speakers. Children who are hearing-impaired can become quite confused by having one language spoken at home and another at school. Parents of such children should be helped to learn English. Manual communication, used either as an alternative to spoken language or in parallel with it, can also limit the extent to which a child can learn to perceive and use spoken language. If verbal learning is considered to be a desirable and reasonable goal, factors which can adversely influence its development must

be restricted or eliminated so that its achievement becomes both feasible and practical.

7. *Abundant interaction between the child and his hearing peers.* That the child should be saturated with normal patterns of speech has been stressed above. Frequent contact of a hearing-impaired child with his hearing peers not only ensures copious exposure to spoken language, but stimulates the child emotionally, socially, and intellectually. Children normally conform much more closely to the patterns of speech and behavior of their peers than to the models provided by the parents or other adults. For example, teachers have much less influence on the speech and language of a child from a ghetto than does his contact with peers. So it is with hearing-impaired children. If hearing-impaired children are placed with others who have impoverished speech and language patterns, their verbal learning will also tend to be impoverished, first, because their experience of normal patterns will be reduced and, second, because they will tend to conform to the abnormal system of communication employed by their peers. Self-contained classes and provision that limits interaction with family and normal-hearing children in out-of-school hours therefore create an additional barrier to spoken language acquisition. If, for a given child, there is no alternative to such provision, then measures to counteract the hazards of placement in a segregated setting must be taken. Such measures as employment of sufficient aides and caretakers to ensure adequate verbal interaction on a one-to-one basis are both more expensive and less satisfactory than arrangements which permit socialization with normal-hearing children.

8. *Adequate support services.* A variety of support services is essential to the efficient function of any form of special educational provision for hearing-impaired children. In addition to regular medical checks, semi-annual examinations by an otologist are required to ensure the prevention (or, if necessary, the treatment) of ear disease that could limit hearing aid usage and/or worsen hearing levels. Children who wear hearing aids are at greater risk of ear disease than others. In the course of routine screening, some 5–10 percent of young children in a regular school population are commonly found to have ear disease that warrants medical attention. In view of the importance of vision in speech reception by severely hearing-impaired children, regular eye examinations are also essential. While occasional support services may be

required of a psychiatrist, psychologist, and social worker, the services of an audiologist and an electronic technician, skilled in hearing aid maintenance, should be continuously available to the hearing-impaired child and his teacher/clinician. Unless such services are available, hearing aids cannot be maintained in working order and the child's full-time use of amplification cannot be realized. An audiologist and an electronic technician can provide adequate services for about 50–75 children. Specialist teacher/clinicians may themselves be considered as support personnel when the hearing-impaired child is placed in regular classes on either a part- or full-time basis. The number of pupils they can cope with will depend on the nature of the program (see Chapter 13) and the extent of the children's handicap.

Students

Many students in Psychology, Education, Audiology, and Speech Pathology seek information about the various fields that may be open to them with further professional training and about the nature of handicaps which they might meet if they decide to pursue professional work in their present areas of study. This text will, hopefully, provide them with a range of insights into the problems of hearing-impaired children and the possibilities of work with them. Students should note that this text is not a comprehensive introduction to the field, in that our emphasis is upon the development of verbal skills and education through the use of spoken language. It does not treat alternative avenues of development and instruction that, given the opportunities we suggest, would be needed only for the minority of hearing-impaired children. Students should be aware that considerable controversy over methods of educating hearing-impaired children has raged for well over a century. But during this period, enormous technological advances have been made. The potential for the type of work that we discuss in this text has increased proportionally. Advances in actual work with hearing-impaired children have failed to keep pace with emerging knowledge from such disciplines as psychology, audiology, speech science, and electronics because teacher/clinicians already working in the field — and even those now being trained — do not have ready access to available information. This book provides access to such information and at the same time indicates to students what the nature of their future involvement with hearing-impaired children could be. No field of human need is more challenging, and in no area of education or therapy can there be more intrinsically interesting work or a greater shortage of adequately qualified personnel.

ANNOTATED BIBLIOGRAPHY

Babbidge, H. D.   *Education of the Deaf.* Washington, D.C.: U.S. Department of Health, Education and Welfare, 1965.

This Report to the Secretary of Health, Education and Welfare by the Babbidge Advisory Committee on the Education of the Deaf is an objective and comprehensive examination of the needs of hearing-impaired children and their special educational treatment in the United States. It presents a balanced report on the situation facing hearing-impaired children, their parents and their teachers, and makes carefully reasoned recommendations for the improvement of services to them. The situation has changed little since the Report was written.

Ewing, A. W. G., and Ewing, E. C.   *Teaching Deaf Children to Talk.* Manchester, England: Manchester University Press, 1964.

In this text, the Ewings present a clear and simple account of how hearing-impaired children can learn to communicate through the use of spoken language. They include several case histories to illustrate their points. The book describes speech, hearing aids, parent guidance strategies, and the types of educational treatment that best lead to the development of effective verbal skills.

Ling, D., Ling, A. H., and Pflaster, G.   Individualized educational programing for hearing-impaired children. *The Volta Review,* 79, 204–230, 1977.

This is an article in which educational provisions, modes of communication, and the competencies required by teacher/clinicians are discussed. A hundred key references are provided for further reading.

Whetnall, E., and Fry, D. B.   *The Deaf Child.* Springfield, Ill.:
  Charles C Thomas, 1971.

Written by an otologist and a phonetician, both concerned with the
medical and educational treatment of hearing-impaired children, this
text describes how residual hearing can be used to develop spoken
language. The authors describe the mechanisms of speech, the causes
and pathologies of deafness, diagnostic and assessment procedures, and
the development of listening skills in hearing-impaired children. Case
histories are provided to support the type of treatment they recommend—treatment that they have studied with numerous children in
experimental and service settings.

2. Communication

Communication is the sharing of information, opinions, thoughts, ideas, or feelings by two or more individuals. For satisfactory communication to occur, both partners must already share a common system or devise one, so that each can understand the other's intent. For the most part, we adopt the forms of communication used by the family, community, and society into which we are born. Should a situation arise in which neither individual knows the other's system, one must learn from the other, or both have to work out a new system. For example, in the case of a person who has had a stroke and has lost the ability to speak, a system can be worked out so that he can respond to questions requiring Yes or No responses by making a movement of which he is capable, such as raising a finger or closing his eyes. Communication systems can be as simple as the one just described or as complex as spoken language.

Speech, Language, and Communication

Human beings communicate with one another principally through *speech,* that is, we express our thoughts in sequences of articulated sounds to which particular meanings have been attached. The relationship between a sound sequence and its meaning is quite arbitrary and varies from one language to another. For example, "burro" means "donkey" in Spanish and "butter" in Italian. Within a language, apart from a few exceptions which are known as homonyms, each sound sequence has a different meaning. The word *language* has been defined as "the entire body of words and sounds employed by any community for intercommunication." There are many, many languages, each of which has a complex system of rules including those for sequencing sounds into words and combining words into sentences. The grammar or syntax of a language describes the general principles and the particular rules underlying its use. As indicated by the derivation of the word "language" from the Latin *lingua,* meaning tongue, its use was formerly restricted to language as spoken (and later written) by man. Current usage has extended its meaning, as evidenced by such expressions as "body language," "sign language," "the language of the bees," "computer language," and so on. While none involves speech, the underlying notion of a rule-governed system of communication is retained.

Although laymen continue to use the words "speech" and "language" as synonyms, professionals working in the field of human communication disorders find it expedient to create a distinction. Thus parents or others (such as regular classroom teachers) unfamiliar with this special usage may be confused when they are informed that a child has "poor speech, but good language." In this context, the word "speech" refers to the manner in which the child articulates (or pronounces) sounds in syllables, words, and sentences. (For further discussion, see Chapter 9.) The term "language" is intended to refer to knowledge of the entire body of rules governing language use. For diagnostic and remedial purposes greater detail is often provided under headings such as "spoken language," "written language," "receptive vocabulary" (words understood), "expressive vocabulary" (words spoken), and so forth. (This topic is treated in more detail in Chapters 3 and 11, which concern development of language.)

Human beings communicate with a variety of systems in addition to spoken or written language. Smoke signals, traffic signals, drums, semaphore, Morse code, sign language, and others are examples. Some, such as Morse code, involve a simple transformation of spoken language. Whatever the system, there has to be an agreed set of rules for their use.

Animal Communication

Human beings are not the only species with a highly developed system of communication. Animals also communicate effectively with one another, utilizing systems of varying complexity to inform others of the location of food, the extent of their territory, the approach of danger, or in performing elaborate courting rituals. These systems may involve auditory, vocal, visual, tactile, and olfactory signals as well as complicated sequences of body movements. Few of these have been clearly delineated.

It was formerly believed that animal and human communication were vastly different. Animal communication was thought to follow rigid patterns determined biologically. The learning of new systems was thought to be impossible, especially those involving symbols (such as human language). Creativity in combining symbols was considered to be beyond their intellectual capabilities.

Current research is breaking down many of these assumptions. Although attempts to teach apes to talk have been unsuccessful, some have been able to learn to communicate with American Sign Language. Others have been taught to manipulate plastic tokens according to a complicated system, and others are able to communicate with a computer. Up to the present time, all animal communication can be considered nonverbal in nature, in the sense that the term "verbal" implies the use of the spoken or written word.

Spoken Language as an Effective Communication System

An effective communication system is one that permits those using it to exchange information with a high degree of ease, flexibility, speed, and accuracy in a wide variety of circumstances. Spoken language appears to meet those conditions.

It requires little or no effort for most of us to talk to one another. We can do it almost without thinking and frequently we do! In contrast, it is markedly harder for most people to express their thoughts and ideas in writing. Spoken language is easy to acquire, as evidenced by the rapidity with which it is mastered by the normal human infant. Indeed, children learn to talk so easily that few people realize just how complex a process it actually is. It was not until the 1960s that the topic began to receive the concerted attention of a large number of linguists and psychologists and that the field of psycholinguistics opened up as a major area of research.

Spoken language is extremely flexible in nature. We can readily adjust its complexity to suit our listener's needs. With an adult native speaker of our language, we presume understanding. In the case of family, friends, or colleagues, with whose backgrounds we are familiar, we are able to select more or less elaborate sentence structures, technical vocabulary, or even switch to a common dialect, should that be more appropriate. When we talk to a young child or someone unfamiliar with the language, we speak in shorter sentences, and employ a more basic vocabulary.

How accurate is spoken language as a communication system? Our intent can usually be conveyed with accuracy and with considerable precision. However, it is open to misinterpretation. Sometimes we do not hear clearly, we suffer a lapse of attention, or our memory of what was said is faulty. To solve the lack of permanence of the spoken word (except when tape-recorded), we tend to use the written form in contractual agreements. The use of written language also allows us to pass on the accumulated knowledge in various fields of learning. Verbal communication, whether spoken or written, permits a high degree of precision which is not possible when using only nonverbal modes. This is not to say that nonverbal modes are unimportant.

Nonverbal Aspects of Communication

Even when talking to one another face to face, we do not depend entirely on a verbal system. In conversation, for example, we are continually aware of one another's reactions, whether verbal or nonverbal. When recounting an incident we expect a response from our listener every now and then, at the very least a nod of agreement. We usually offer our partner the opportunity to take his turn in the conversation, either verbally—perhaps by asking "And what do you think?"—or nonverbally by pausing and looking toward him for a comment.

Sometimes we are at a loss to express our feelings adequately in words. Our attitudes and feelings are mainly conveyed nonverbally, by means of a glance, a smile or a groan, by turning toward or away from someone, by physical contact, or tone of voice. A person's sincerity may be doubted should his nonverbal expression but weakly reflect his words. Young children are particularly sensitive to nonverbal cues and will tend to react to the latter rather than spoken words when there appears to be conflict.

Nonverbal cues may, of course, be used quite deliberately to alter the literal meaning of a statement. One's facial expression and tone of voice can determine the meaning of the sentence, "I just adore animals." In general, however, nonverbal cues support and therefore facilitate comprehension of spoken language and, as mentioned in Chapter 8, they are especially helpful to hearing-impaired people.

Breakdown of Communication

Indicators of breakdown of communication may be either verbal or nonverbal, direct or indirect. For example, a member of an audience may raise his hand and inform a lecturer that he cannot be heard at the back of the hall. Alternatively, the lecturer himself may notice that members of the audience are leaning forward and cupping their ears and respond to those indirect nonverbal cues by raising his voice or using a microphone and asking the audience directly if he can be heard adequately.

Of course, the effectiveness of any communication system depends basically on the desire and willingness of the persons involved to understand what each is attempting to convey to the other. The consequences of unsatisfactory communication over a long period of time can be quite devastating, both emotionally and socially.

Emotional and Social Aspects of Communication

Men, women, children, and infants are basically social beings and depend on human interaction and companionship for survival. Solitary confinement for a prolonged period usually leads to a breakdown in personality. Infants in institutional settings have been known to become apathetic and depressed through lack of social contact, to lose interest in living, and even to die. Somewhat less dramatic but no less important consequences occur when infants, children, or adults either never acquire or for some reason lose their ability to communicate with their family, friends, workmates, or other social contacts.

In order to feel comfortable and at home in a community, one needs to be familiar with both the verbal and nonverbal aspects of the communication system used by the majority of its members. Those who are not fully conversant with the language and social customs are likely to be or feel themselves to be misunderstood, neglected, or even rejected by society. One's sense of identity may be disturbed if others mock one's accent, dialect, lack of fluency, or even manner of dress. Reactions to being or feeling to be a social misfit may include becoming passive and withdrawn, or alternatively hostile and destructive.

Hearing Impairment and Communication

The effects that hearing impairment has upon communication depend on a variety of factors, including the degree of hearing impairment, age at onset of the problem, and the timing and type of (re)habilitation treatment provided.

Degree of Hearing Impairment

Hearing impairment can range in severity from a mild defect that goes unnoticed to a total loss of auditory function. Mild hearing defects are extremely common and most people suffer from them either occasionally, as during a cold, or permanently, as is the case with teenagers who have destroyed some of their sensory nerve cells through listening to popular music at very high levels of intensity. Mild hearing impairments of either type may have no significant effect on communication. Indeed, slight hearing loss can be tolerated because most of us have more hearing than we really need. Hearing is normally so acute that whispered conversation can be heard over substantial distances. Such sensitivity is not essential to learning or using spoken language.

People who may be considered as having moderate hearing impairment are those who can hear speech clearly when they are in one-to-one communication with others at close quarters, but cannot hear speech distinctly under most other circumstances. In older people, such hearing impairment often leads to their listening to television or radio at somewhat higher-than-normal levels of intensity and to complaints that "everybody seems to mumble these days." This problem is due to the fact that some sounds of speech, such as vowels, are much louder than others, such as the consonants [f] and [s]. Speech appears to be indistinct to those with moderate hearing impairment because the louder sounds are clearly audible while the quieter sounds are not (see Chapter 4). Many adults with moderate hearing difficulties would rather cherish the illusion that they have no problem than seek treatment for it. In doing so, they may impose quite a burden upon those with whom they are in contact. Treatment for moderate hearing impairment is often sought by the elderly at the instigation of others, usually family members who find it hard to live with someone who makes them raise their voices or suffer accusations like "You're talking about me behind my back."

Severe hearing impairment may be said to exist when little or no speech can be heard even in a one-to-one situation. When audition is so limited, communication through speech is well nigh impossible unless speechreading (lipreading) is used and/or a hearing aid is worn. One cannot deal with such a problem just by speaking at louder-than-normal levels. People with severe hearing problems cannot follow programs on the television or radio simply by turning up the volume. Even the most suitable hearing aids may not render all speech sounds audible to a person with severe hearing impairment. Even so, they can usually restore ability to communicate to adults who have previously been able to hear. Such persons are familiar with what people are likely to say in certain social situations and they are so familiar with their language that they are in a position to predict a large amount of what might be said. They can also reconstruct sentences that are predicted inaccurately or partly missed by holding the words or sounds they did hear in memory and scanning back to make sense of these fragments. The ability of adults to use very limited auditory cues in this way can be illustrated by asking someone to identify a nursery rhyme, simply from the rhythm of its words tapped out on a table.

Age at Onset

Moderate or severe hearing impairment is a much more serious problem for children than for adults who once heard normally. Children do not have the social, speech, language, or verbal memory skills that help so much in the interpretation of partial auditory patterns. Those who are born with such hearing impairment have to learn these skills before they can communicate verbally and with ease. Those who become hearing-impaired during childhood have some advantages over children born with the problem, but not so many advantages as the adult who suffers loss of hearing.

Children born with moderate hearing impairment usually acquire limited speech communication skills because many of the voiced sounds of speech, including those they themselves produce, will be audible to them. They will, however, fail to hear the unvoiced sounds of speech and most conversation at a distance will not reach them. Accordingly, their speech will be faulty and their language development will be delayed unless their hearing impairment is quickly recognized and treated.

All speech is inaudible to those who are severely hearing-impaired unless hearing aids are worn. Even then, certain patterns may be imperceptible. Children born with a severe hearing deficit can not, therefore, learn to communicate verbally without special help. Initially, like all other children, they will vocalize, but such vocalization—which is reflex in nature—will not develop into speech unless habilitation is begun early in life (see Chapter 10).

Children who suffer severe loss of hearing after they have acquired spoken language may lose their communication skills unless they receive specialist treatment immediately. If delay in treatment is allowed to occur, previously acquired communication skills may be wholly or partly lost. Loss of such skills is more rapid among younger than among older children, simply because younger children have had less opportunity to practice them. In order to maintain communication skills, children must learn to interpret whatever acoustic information they can receive through hearing aids, learn speechreading skills, and maintain control of their articulation of speech through compensatory mechanisms. If delay is avoided, their previous verbal experience can help them to communicate normally in spite of their hearing loss, since they have the same skills—albeit less well established—as those described for adults.

Total deafness is rare either at birth or as a result of childhood illness. The totally deaf child has only two senses available for speech reception: vision and touch. Neither sense is particularly well suited for the task. Speech reception skills are therefore hard (but not impossible) for a born-deaf child to learn. Only limited and ambiguous patterns are available through speechreading, but these can be sufficient for speech reception when contextual cues are provided. Touch, together with vision, can provide enough information for the development of intelligible speech (see Chapters 8 and 9). Children who suffer complete loss of hearing after having acquired language can usually learn to compensate sufficiently for such loss by using vision and touch, and continue to communicate normally. Verbal communication with totally deaf persons, whether they were born without hearing or acquired deafness later in life, is rarely effortless.

Habilitation Treatment

The type of habilitation provided for hearing-impaired children will largely determine how well they acquire verbal communication skills. The more severe the hearing impairment; the earlier its onset; and the later treatment is begun, all make more necessary carefully structured training. Hearing impairment is a serious barrier to verbal learning, and with those whose hearing impairment is more than minimal, it can only be gained through deliberate programming. Our approach to such programming is described in the following chapters.

ANNOTATED BIBLIOGRAPHY

Laver, J., and Hutcheson, S. (Eds.)   *Communication in Face to Face Interaction.* Harmondsworth, Middlesex, Eng.: Penguin Books, 1972.
This inexpensive paperback contains a selection of papers by well-known authors, dating back to Sapir (1927). The emphasis is on such nonverbal aspects of human communication as gaze direction, body language, voice characteristics, and the use of personal space.

Miller, G. A. (Ed.)   *Communication, Language, and Meaning: Psychological Perspectives.* New York: Basic Books, 1973.
Suitable for the layman or beginning student, this book provides a broad coverage of topics, each written by an expert. The material was initially presented in the form of broadcast talks on The Voice of America.

Wood, B. S.   *Children and Communication: Verbal and Nonverbal Language Development.* Englewood Cliffs, N.J.: Prentice-Hall, 1976.
This book is concerned with verbal and nonverbal aspects of communication from infancy to adolescence. Body language, proxemics (distance between speakers), and prosodic features are discussed.

3. Development of Spoken Language

*I*n the brief span of three to four years, the normally developing infant progresses from a gross, largely undifferentiated
form of communication (crying versus non-crying) to a highly
refined system corresponding fairly closely to that used by the
adults in his immediate family circle. Normally, a baby produces
his first clear words around the time of his first birthday, uses
two-word phrases when he is 2, and talks in short sentences by the
time he is 3.

By the age of 3 or 4 years, most children are able to express
themselves fluently in their native or mother tongue. They are
able to understand most of what is said to them and can communicate their needs, wants, and ideas to even strangers. By age
5, they are in a position to benefit from formal schooling since
they have access to the common code, spoken language, in which
instruction is provided. Initial teaching and a considerable portion of all later instruction are conveyed through speech.

Because children understand the language spoken around
them, they are also able to learn incidentally. Consequently, they
absorb the moral, social, cultural, and educational values of the
community in which they live through an interaction of example
and the spoken word. Providing they observe these values, they
will be accepted as integral members of that community.

The Search for Knowledge on Language Acquisition

During the 1960s, psycholinguists focused on the child's acquisition of syntax. They seemed to view the onset of language as the
point at which a child frequently combined two words to form

phrases. In the early 1970s, the emphasis began to shift from grammatical to semantic aspects of early two-word phrases. By observing the situation in which a child uttered a phrase such as "Daddy . . . car," one could determine whether he was conveying the notion of possession (That's Daddy's car) rather than location (Daddy's in the car).

Interest then turned to tracing the process by which the child's expressive language developed from single word utterances to the use of words in a sequence. The notion that the child's ability to combine words might depend on his having developed certain cognitive concepts is currently being studied.

In spite of this trend to perceive a developmental progression in language acquisition, linguists—apart from some notable exceptions—have generally rejected the notion that there is continuity of development from the early speech sounds through to their use as carriers of the spoken language. It is our view that the intimate knowledge of the phonetic repertoire of his language gained through extended periods of listening and babbling must be of major help to the infant in the formidable task of decoding the language spoken around him.

The Nature of Language

The nature of language is so complicated that several distinct fields of study have emerged. The major areas are *phonology, semantics,* and *syntax.* Phonology involves the study of speech sounds as they are used in the language; semantics is concerned with the meanings of the sound patterns (both words and sentences) of the language; and syntax is the body of rules by which words are combined to form sentences.

Phonology

Native mastery of the phonologic aspects of a language include accurate perception and production of its phonemes (see Chapter 4), ability to produce and modify them in fluent speech, and the appropriate use of suprasegmental patterns (pitch, stress, intonation). It also includes the ability to recognize sound patterns which are not part of the language, but could be adopted as a new word as compared with one which could not. For example, [tas]* would be acceptable as an English word, but not [tsa]. Knowledge of the

*The key to the phonetic spellings is shown on page vi

phonology would also permit one to figure out the probable pronunciation of a word first encountered in its written form.

Semantics

The words of a language consist of particular sequences of
sounds to which particular meanings have become associated over
a period of time. We learn to attend to small differences between
sound patterns because they convey different meanings, for
example [pat] and [tap], [pat] and [pɛt], [splɪt] and [spɪlt]. Most
words have multiple related meanings.

Sometimes a particular sound sequence has two distinctly different meanings. Such words are known as homonyms. For
example, [rɛd] can either be a color, or the past tense of the verb
"to read." The linguistic context resolves the ambiguity, thus "I
have red shoes" and "I have read the notice." This feature of
spoken language leads to both unintentional and deliberate
humorous effects such as puns. Native users of a language are
familiar with synonyms which are words with quite different pronunciation but similar, though rarely exactly the same, meanings.
Synonomous expressions can also be found for sentences. The
semantic content of a paragraph is retained when it is para-
phrased, as is that of a book when it is condensed.

Knowing the meaning of the individual words in a sentence is
not sufficient to enable one to understand idiomatic expressions.
These phrases have to be learned, in the appropriate context, as
complete units. Attempts at literal translation of idioms from one
language to another are likely to amuse or bewilder the listener
unless he is familiar with both languages.

Within the area of semantics, morphology has been defined as
the study of minimal units of meaning. These units, or morphemes, can be words or parts of words, such as suffixes, prefixes,
or inflections which denote plurals, possessives, verb tense, and
subject-verb agreement. For example, the word "smaller" consists
of two morphemes, namely "small" and "-er". Other examples of
words divided into morphemes are walk-ed; farm-er; un-reason-
able. Certain words do not fit the definition of morpheme since
they do not by themselves convey meaning. These words, such as
"for," "to," "by," and "it," have an important function in sentences
and for this reason are known as "functors" or function words.

A native speaker's intuitive knowledge of his language leads
him to inflect new words according to the morphological rules.

For example, if he hears that a "fitch" has been purchased by the local zoo, he would know that if they bought another, there would be two "fitches." Similarly, he would deduce that the past tense of "He is fitching" would be "He fitched." This aspect of language is acquired naturally and does not depend on formal teaching.

Syntax

Knowledge of the syntactic rules of a language is necessary for the comprehension and construction of statements and questions, for the use of negatives, passives, subjunctives, auxiliary verbs, verb tenses, pronouns, relative clauses, and so on. Most of this knowledge is acquired spontaneously by the young child before he goes to school. No native speaker of a language experiences any difficulty (barring the finer points of grammar) in identifying which are, and which are not, acceptable sentences. For example, "He went for a walk" is an acceptable English sentence, whereas "He for a walk went" is not. Pseudo-sentences can be constructed that are syntactically correct, in that they obey the rules of grammar, but are semantically inappropriate and therefore meaningless. An example is "The rotated germs enraged the hopeful milk."

Theories of Language Acquisition

Given the complexity of spoken languages, and the difficulty that most of us, as adults, experience in trying to learn a second language, how is it that the majority of children achieve basic mastery of their native tongue as easily as they do?

One common viewpoint has been that language is essentially learned through imitation and reinforcement. The baby accidentally produces sounds, such as "dada" or "mama," which are then imitated and reinforced by the parents. Parents then teach the child names of objects by pointing to the object, saying its name, and encouraging the child to repeat it. A similar tactic is presumably employed with phrases and sentences. This theory does not account for the young child's ability to understand a wide range of sentences he has never heard before, nor does it show how he can create sentences of his own that he has never heard others produce. Although the processes of imitation and reinforcement may be neither necessary nor sufficient in themselves to explain how language is acquired, they do normally play a considerable part in language acquisition.

In contrast to those who support the view that language is learned behavior, there are those who believe that the child is born with a mechanism which permits him to deduce all the phonologic, semantic, and syntactic rules of the particular language to which he is exposed as an infant. Exactly how such an innate language acquisition device works is far from clear. What does seem to be clear is that the human brain is specially equipped to process spoken language. Research undertaken with normal and brain-injured subjects shows that, for most of us, it is the left hemisphere which has this function, the right hemisphere being more involved with nonverbal, spatial, wholistic processing. Damage to the left hemisphere in adult life usually results in paralysis of the right side of the body along with disruption of the person's ability to comprehend and produce language. Recovery of language skills is both slow and uncertain. Should damage occur to the language areas of the brain in early childhood, it appears that other areas of the brain can often take over, and recovery of language function is rapid. Such plasticity has been thought to be possible because of incomplete specialization.

Until relatively recently, it was believed that the two hemispheres of the infant brain had equal potential for development and that it was only gradually, over the first five or six years, that certain areas of the brain became specialized. More recent research indicates that hemispheric specialization is present at birth.

Barriers to Language Development

Language can be acquired in spite of many problems. Severe mental retardation greatly delays—but does not prevent—language acquisition, providing that the child is not secluded from contact with those who talk. Neither does the inability to articulate the sounds of speech prevent a child from learning to understand what is said. Although unable to see what is being referred to, the young blind child can learn to associate the auditory patterns with the impressions gained through his other senses. He has relatively minor problems in language acquisition.

Deafness from infancy is probably the greatest barrier to the development of any language which is based on the spoken form. Contrary to what might be thought, language is not readily learned through the written form. This topic will be discussed in Chapters 11 and 12.

Language as an Auditory Code

Access to the special linguistic processor of the brain is direct through the auditory modality. The nature of language is intrinsically based on differences between sound patterns and learning the meanings which are arbitrarily associated with them.

Those who are unable to differentiate any sound patterns are faced with the extraordinarily difficult task of painstakingly learning to associate visible movements of the lips, jaw, and tongue with meanings. Learning a language through speechreading is enormously harder than learning to speechread a language that was acquired through hearing (see Chapter 8).

Echoic memory permits brief storage of incoming auditory patterns to be compared and contrasted with those already stored in long-term memory. The suprasegmental aspects—duration, loudness and pitch—of the spoken form add richness and color to the phonetic character of the signal, making it more likely to be remembered than would be evenly stressed syllables spoken in a monotone. The normal, rhythmic patterns of speech group words together to make phrases which are perceived as meaningful units. The child with normal hearing does not have to analyze the spoken message phoneme by phoneme, and word by word, in order to discover its meaning. In the beginning, he is likely to understand certain phrases as a whole, for example, "Don't-touch," "Put-it-back," "There-it-is," without any awareness of the boundaries between the words.

Skills Relevant to Spoken Language

By the end of his first year of life, the baby has developed many skills which are essential for effective speech communication.

Social Interaction

The year-old baby has learned a great deal about how to gain and maintain the attention of others. He initiates communication by vocalizing, laughing and shouting, by making eye contact and then smiling, by touching and tugging. He responds when others approach him. He turns around when called and looks at people when they talk to him. He smiles and vocalizes in response to speech. He takes turns in "conversations." He plays "pat-a-cake" and "peek-a-boo." He knows his parents, siblings, and others who spend much time with him; he may be wary of strangers.

Auditory Perception and Memory

The year-old baby is able, and has been almost from birth, to discriminate quite fine differences between speech sounds (for example, between [pa], [ta] and [ka], between [ba] and [ma], and between vowels). Even the one-month-old infant has sufficient auditory memory capacity to hear a sequence of repeated syllables, such as [papapa . . .], and retain it for sufficient time to compare and differentiate it from an immediately following sequence, such as [tatata . . .]. The baby can associate a variety of non-speech sounds with meaning, the clink of saucepans indicating preparation of food, the bark of the family dog, the sounds of his toy musical box and rattle, the sound of footsteps indicating that someone is coming. He also links voices with people. By the end of the first year, he appears to be attuned to the sound patterns of the language around him, and may become very quiet and attentive when he hears a foreign language.

Auditory-Vocal Feedback

The baby has learned to integrate hearing and speech. By listening to his own and others' vocalizations, he has learned to produce a wide variety of sounds, including some special effects, and he can imitate vowels or syllables which are already in his repertoire.

Motor-Speech Skills

The year-old child has developed sufficient control over his speech musculature so that, at will, he can produce long or short utterances and can vary the pitch and loudness of his voice. He can produce long strings of syllables, repeated ones such as [dadada] and alternated or varied ones such as [gagigu]. His vocal repertoire might allow one to guess which language he hears around him, be it English, French or Chinese.

Understanding and Using Meaningful Voice Patterns

Before the child is capable of understanding speech, he is able to derive meaning from voice patterns. A quiet, soothing voice indicates that comfort is at hand, whereas a loud, sharp voice, perhaps directed at a sibling, may be a warning to stop ongoing activity. Before he is able to talk, the baby can express his anger or pleasure by varying the pitch, duration, and loudness of his voice. He may say "oh oh" to indicate "Oh, I've dropped my spoon."

He seems to understand that a rising intonation pattern followed by a pause (a question), requires that he respond. His own first attempts at asking questions consist of a mixture of vocal and nonverbal components. For example, he will seek permission for some previously forbidden activity, such as switching on the television, by making eye contact with his mother and vocalizing. Then, as he is about to touch it, he will look toward his mother and vocalize again, perhaps with a rising intonation pattern, as much as to say "okay?"

Understanding the Situation

The child has also learned to interpret the ongoing situation and knows the sequence of routine events. He can predict what is about to happen on the basis of his memory of past experiences. Thus, when he sees his mother putting on her coat and picking up her purse, without having dressed him in his outdoor clothes, he concludes that he is going to be left behind, and protests loudly. Activity in the kitchen indicates the approach of mealtime, and the running of bath water, that soon he can splash and play with his toy ducks.

Concepts

The child has acquired many important notions and concepts on the basis of his sensory-motor experience. For example, he is aware of himself as a being existing in his own right, able to control many of his own actions and, to some extent, the actions of others. He has developed notions relating to the permanence of objects. He knows that his toys continue to exist even when he cannot see them and that if he looks for them, he may be able to find them. He has learned to point and vocalize to indicate a desired object or to draw someone's attention to an interesting event or activity.

Symbolization

The ability to symbolize is a major advance in cognitive development. It is first evidenced, usually at about the age of 10 months, in the child's consistent use of a gesture to signify a particular idea. He adopts the conventions of his culture. For example, he shakes his head when he doesn't want to do something and he waves his hand when he is about to leave the room.

At this point in development, communication could evolve in

the form of an increasingly elaborate system of gestures, such as the conventional sign language used by communities of deaf people. Instead of learning such a visual-gestural system, most children are exposed to an auditory-verbal system in which objects, actions, and ideas are represented by particular phonetic patterns. Perhaps in an attempt to facilitate the baby's initiation into the language of his community, some of his own babble patterns are used as names for his mother and father. The actual phonetic patterns vary from one language to another. In English, these are [mama] and [dada], later changing to "mommy" and "daddy," or "mom" and "dad."

Comprehension and Use of Spoken Language

Toward the end of the first year of life, there seems to be a converging force in operation. The baby becomes increasingly able to integrate all the skills we have described and begins to apply them toward the mastery of spoken language.

The baby applies his knowledge of a situation, together with his understanding of voice patterns and facial expression, to help him figure out the meaning of the language addressed to him. As his locomotor skills develop, he begins to explore his home environment. He opens and shuts cupboard doors, he climbs on low chairs or tables, he smells and tastes everything. Because of his compulsion to touch everything, he soon learns the meaning of phrases such as "Don't touch" and "That's hot," and the consequences of ignoring them. In addition to vivid experiences which leave a strong impression in his memory, the child's daily routine of bathing, feeding, dressing, and diapering offers many occasions for the gradual association of spoken phrases with their accustomed meaning.

The child's auditory perceptual skills make it easy for him to differentiate the varied sound patterns he hears. His ability to produce many of the phonetic and suprasegmental aspects of the language spoken around him must surely assist him in remembering the correspondence of sound patterns and their meanings. When asked, "Do you want a banana?" and shown one, he is likely to mimic [nana]. Since [nana] is one of his own familiar babble patterns, he is likely to remember what it refers to, and may recognize the word "banana" next time he hears it spoken. If later, he says [nana] as he points to a banana, his utterance is likely to be interpreted as a word approximation, and his mother may say "Yes, that's a banana." On another occasion, he may say [nana], without seeing a banana, and his mother may then check his intended reference by asking him if he wants a banana.

Words which are not part of the baby's babble repertoire (e.g. "drink") may be more difficult for him to remember and attach to a meaning. However, if a particular word or phrase occurs often enough in routine situations, and in such a way that its reference is clear, the baby will come to recognize it. Several weeks, of course, may pass before he is able to retrieve the pattern from memory and produce a recognizable approximation. Those who have attempted learning a second language as an adult should be familiar with the experience.

Perhaps because people are so important to him, the baby learns very early the spoken patterns which are used to identify them. By the age of 12 months or so, he can point correctly when asked "Where's Mommy?" or "Where's Daddy?" He knows his own name and alerts to it instantly. He recognizes the names of his siblings and anyone else who spends a lot of time with him.

Parental Role in Language Learning

The baby learning his native language is in a much more fortunate position than an adult learning a foreign language. The expectations are much less, for the baby's every attempt to talk is liberally rewarded. Even a gross approximation, such as /ɪ/ or /dɪ/ for "drink," is accepted. His "baby" words are considered cute. Without special teaching, but as and when he is able, the baby improves his approximation to "ding" or "dink." Only when parents feel it to be socially important do they pressure their child to speak, for example, "hi," "bye-bye," "please" and "thank you."

Parents, other adults, and older children seem to adapt their speech and language patterns automatically when talking to little children. The adult learning a foreign language is rarely accommodated to in this way. Conversation between adults is frequently disjointed. The topic is changed without warning. A great deal is taken for granted. When speaking to a baby, short simple phrases, clearly relevant to the immediate situation, are used. The baby is spoken to directly, in a one-to-one situation, and is not expected to understand rapid speech addressed to others. Cues to the verbal message are supplied liberally in the form of somewhat exaggerated intonation patterns and facial expression.

A shared activity frequently forms the focus of such verbal interaction. For example, the baby's father might build up a tower of blocks saying, "Let's build up the blocks. Up they go. Up, up, up, up." Then, as the baby starts to knock them down, his father may say, "Knock them down. Down they go. Down." As the baby laughs and indicates that he wants a repeat performance, father may say, "Shall we do it again? Okay, build them up, up, up," etc. The baby's delight in playing the same game over and over encourages the adult to provide the child with the verbal repetition required for language learning.

Between the age of 10 and 15 months, the baby progresses from a complete absence of verbal comprehension to the stage where he has a small receptive vocabulary of words and phrases which he is able to understand without situational or other cues. He recognizes these words even when they occur in adult conversation. Thus, the mere mention of the word "bed" or "sleep" will bring howls of protest, whereas the word "car" will be echoed, while he trots delightedly toward the door in anticipation of a car ride.

First Words and Their Meanings

The young child's early word approximations have their own field of meaning. For example, /ka/ may initially be used in a restricted sense, referring only to the family car. Shortly thereafter its use may be extended, as it was by our elder son, Philip, at age 12 months, to refer not only to other cars, but to trucks, buses, vans, and even bicycles. He had apparently perceived all of these as having sufficient in common to be given the same label. This particular usage lasted a very short time, probably because he was told, "That's not a car. It's a truck." or "That's a bike." Before long he began to use /rʌ/ for "truck" and /baɪ/ for "bike." Such over-extension in the early use of words may be related to perceptual features of the objects, such as their shape, size, taste, texture, or movement.

The young child may use a particular sound pattern to represent several different objects, not because he is confused about their names, but simply because he is unable to pronounce the words in an adult fashion. Thus, he may resort to using /bʌ/ for *brush, button, butter* and *bucket,* all of which he has in his receptive vocabulary. Since the situation generally resolves the potential ambiguity, the child's approximations will be accepted. As his motor-speech skills improve, he will produce distinctly different approximations, such as/bʌʃ/for "brush" and /bʌnɪ /for "button."

Another problem that arises in early word acquisition is the case of mistaken reference. An example of this occurred with Philip at age 13 months. He used /tiθ/, first in association with the act of brushing his teeth, then in reference to his toothbrush, next his hairbrush, then any other brush. Finally, at 15 months, he said /brʌ/ for "brush" and thereafter used /tiθ/ for "teeth" in the accepted way.

The child's appreciation of words and their meanings is often a reflection of his conceptual knowledge. The 18-month-old who uses the words "big" and "heavy" interchangeably does so understandably, since to him most big objects are heavy, and most heavy things, big. The 21-month-old who comments on the sudden appearance of the moon with "Oh-oh, light on," no doubt draws on his knowledge that lights can be switched off and on. The process of word acquisition and refinement of meanings continues not only throughout childhood but also in adult life.

Growth of Spoken Vocabulary

The child's spoken vocabulary increases much more slowly than his receptive vocabulary, as a rule. At the age of 16 or 17 months he may give clear evidence of understanding as many as 30 or 40 words, while using only a few word approximations. For example, he might know words such as "juice," "milk," "cookie," "candy," "bath," "bed," "shoes," "coat," "ball," etc., yet use only four or five words such as "mommy," "daddy," "up," "no," "mo(re)," "hot." Babble sounds such as [dɪdɪ] and [ʌ ʌ], accompanied by pointing, may be used to indicate food and drink, or indeed anything he wants.

As mentioned earlier, the child's first word approximations are usually single vowels, /ɛ/ for "egg," single syllables, /tɛ/ for "teddy" or repeated syllables, /nana/ for "banana." The next step is to add initial or final consonants or to increase the number of syllables. Thus, the progression for the word "apple" might be /æ/ at 12 months, /æp̄/ at 13 months, /æpə/ at 14 months, normal pronunciation not being achieved till age 2. Another example illustrates the variants used by our younger son, Alister, for the word "cookie." It was pronounced correctly at 14 months, then /tʊtɪ/ and /tʊkɪ/ were used interchangeably until the correct form was reinstated at

20 months. In his early approximations to polysyllabic words or expressions, the baby may reproduce only the vowels, such as /eɪɪ/ for "there-it-is," as did Alister at 16 months, the consonants being filled in weeks or months later.

It is easy to see why the gap between receptive and expressive vocabulary is great in some children. In some cases, the baby's every wish is anticipated, and he has no need to learn the language of his community. In others, the baby is very engrossed in developing his locomotor skills. Sometimes there is insufficient social interaction. In other cases, the child may be unable to match what he says with what he hears, and jargon results.

Sooner or later, there is a turning point characterized by the young child becoming very alert when people talk to him and frequently echoing fairly clearly something of what they say. He may suddenly become aware that things have names and that using those names makes it easier to get what he wants—or at least to ensure that others know what he wants. He not only imitates what others say, he begins to ask what things are called. "Wazzat?" he says, no sooner getting an answer than he points to something else. The young child often continues to ask for the names of objects he already knows, possibly because he wants to check if his memory of the spoken pattern is correct, or possibly because he is not sure whether this particular example can share the same label. He may want to verify that a picture of an object has the same name as the actual object. This type of verbal game, initiated by the child or by his mother, constitutes a worthwhile learning experience. It is often continued by the child when looking at books or playing by himself.

Just how much repetition is required before a child either understands or uses a word or phrase? In some cases, there may have been thousands of repetitions; in others, because of the drama of the situation, once may be enough. A great deal of repetition is probably necessary in the learning of first words, but once the child is able to mimic the adult's pattern with some facility, he may hear a new word and begin to use it immediately. An example of this occurred with Philip, then aged about 16 months. We were driving along a highway and saw many giant pylons carrying electric cables across the country. "Wazzat?" he asked. "That's a pylon," he was told. He then proceeded to name each pylon we passed. "Pylon. Pylon. That a pylon. See pylon, mummy?" In this fashion, Philip rehearsed the word, probably about 50 times, as we drove along over the next several miles.

Rate of Vocabulary Growth

The child's vocabulary seems to grow at a logarithmic rate. Accurate counts of a child's total vocabulary, either receptive or expressive, are hard to obtain. Figures quoted in the literature are usually estimates and they vary considerably from one authority to another. The results of an actual count of spoken vocabulary are shown, for three boys, in Table 3.A. In each case, the child's words (or word approximations) were noted down by his mother. Such tracking of expressive vocabulary allows for a fairly complete inventory for the single word stage, especially when it is undertaken by someone who is with the child during most of his waking hours. In tracing the early development of receptive vocabulary, words and phrases commonly spoken to the child were listed and his ability to comprehend them, without cue, was noted. Beyond the single word stage, the strategy used was to work from a vocabulary list, checking those understood without cue, and adding others known to the child, but not on the list. These data show that the growth rate of vocabulary differs markedly from one child to the next, and in the same child, from one time to another.

TABLE 3.A
A SPOKEN VOCABULARY COUNT UNDERTAKEN
ON 3 BOYS

Figures for the first 2,000 words of **receptive** vocabulary appear in parentheses. The onset of abundant connected speech precluded accurate word-by-word count of *expressive* vocabulary.

Child	\	\	\	\	\	Age in Months	\	\	\	\	\	\
	12	13	14	15	16	17	18	20	21	24	30	36
Martin	3	4	5	7	9	15	49	99*	210	------		
					(42)		(650)					(2000+)
Philip	4	38	80*	110	------							
	(17)	(69)	(105)				(863)			(2000+)		
Alister	3	8	31	61	86	138*	280	------				
	(12)	(32)	(62)	(88)			(360)			(1200)	(1500)	(2000+)

* 2-word phrases common
------Abundant connected speech

The growth of spoken vocabulary is, we believe, accelerated if the child is able to articulate clearly. The child who is able to imitate words (and phrases) fairly accurately would seem to have an enormous advantage over the child with poor articulation. The child who produces recognizable words and phrases receives lots of reinforcement, since his wants are readily understood. His own well-articulated patterns also allow for easy referral and retrieval from long-term memory.

Some Semantic and Syntactic Aspects of Early Language

The child's early vocabulary is by no means restricted to names of things. Indeed, it frequently includes approximations to words such as *up, down, in, out, on, off, again, more, all-gone, hot, dirty, no,* and *me.* These words have considerable power in enabling the child to communicate where he wants to go (up, down, in, out, here, there), what he wants to do (take some article of clothing off or put it on), what he is experiencing (hot, dirty), what he wants (more) and what he doesn't want (no). Thus even at the single word stage, the young child is able to express semantic categories such as object names, location, possession, attribution (description), action, and negation.

Primitive syntactic functions also appear. The young child uses rising intonation to indicate that he's asking permission, "Up?", as opposed to a loud flat or falling pattern, "Up!", which is intended as an order. While still at the single word stage, some morphological rules are applied. His concepts of plurality and possession are now expressed linguistically as in "books," "boys" or "Mommy's," "Daddy's." This requires fairly precise articulation. As he adds words to his vocabulary, he does not always use the appropriate phonologic form /-s, -z or -əz/.

Included in the young child's vocabulary at this stage are approximations to phrases such as "put-it-back," "all-gone," "there-it-is," "open it," and "bad-boy." The child is quite unaware of word boundaries. With experience, he learns that there are "good boys" as well as "bad boys" and "bad girls," and he lets it be known that there are "bad Mummys," too! This example of deliberate combining and recombining of words to create his own phrases is characteristic of the next major development, which usually occurs around 21 months of age. The construction of phrases probably depends on certain minimum cognitive abilities, in that unless the child is able to handle relationships between ideas, he will not be able to express them linguistically. However, the absence of word combinations cannot be regarded as an index of intelligence.

Constructing Phrases

The child's first attempts at putting words together sound rather disjointed, each word being followed by a pause. He says "boat . . . Daddy," "knee . . . Mommy" and is understood only by those present who are able to see that he wants to go out in the boat with Daddy, or that he is in the process of climbing onto Mommy's knee. Word order tends to be variable. He is as likely to say "candy . . . more," as "more candy." Sometimes he seems to state the main idea first and then comment on it.

As his vocabulary becomes less sparse, the young child elaborates. Instead of baldly stating "cat," he may say "big cat" or "cat all-gone"; instead of "no," he says "no bed"; instead of "in," he specifies "in car"; instead of simply demanding "more," he says "more candy." He clearly indicates both the possessor and the possession, "my book," "Mummy's coat."

An important advance is the child's verbal expression of the semantic relationship between actor and action, and between action and object. Thus, when he sees his father kick a ball, instead of the earlier, loosely related words, "Daddy . . . ball," the child now says "Daddy kick" (actor + action) or "kick ball" (action + object). The component parts of a grammatical sentence have begun to emerge.

The combination of the three key elements, actor, action and object (in semantic terms), or subject, verb, object (in grammatical terms), in a single utterance follows some time later and permits verbal communication of a much higher quality. When the child can produce a primitive or "kernel" sentence such as "Daddy kick ball," he need hardly rely on the non-verbal aspects of the situation to convey his ideas. The rest is refinement and occurs with astonishing rapidity, so that by the age of 3 or 4 years, the child has clearly mastered the basic skills of his native language.

Imitation and Creativity

Whether immediate or delayed, vocal or subvocal, imitation is undeniably useful in acquiring a large vocabulary of spoken words. To what extent can it contribute to syntactic development? Present-day linguists doubt whether imitation has any role whatsoever. Our view is that imitation has a small, but nevertheless useful, part to play. All-day interaction with young children who are actually in the process of language acquisition permits parents, and in particular the mother, to know what phrases and sentences are frequently used in the child's presence and are part of his daily routine. It is then possible to identify phrases which may have been memorized, rather than created (e.g., *Don't knock it down! Don't do that!*). For the child to imitate a sentence readily, its length and syntactic complexity must resemble his current spontaneous production. More often, the child will reproduce only a part of a phrase or sentence he has heard, usually the words which are more heavily stressed and which occur toward the end of the sentence. Thus, if his mother asks, "Shall we go in the car?", he may reply "Go car." An example of delayed imitation would be Alister's spontaneous use, at 2 years 4 months, of "I back in minute." The extent to which partial or reduced forms of imitation are used seems to vary widely from child to child.

The child's imitative ability seems to parallel his linguistic ability. In order to memorize lengthy rhymes, jingles and stories, he has to be familiar with much of the vocabulary and syntactic structures involved. Some words he may not understand. Initially, he may only fill in the last word in a line, e.g., "Jack and Jill went up the _____ ." Later, he may reproduce longer phrases such as "Who be sleeping in my bed?", with appropriate voice and intonation patterns. The young child's inability to handle the linguistic structure of the model he is attempting to imitate is shown by the following example. Philip, age 4 years 8 months, said "We're going to sleep on all these cushions," to which his brother Alister (2 years 10 months) responded, "We going to sleep on these cush, on these all cushions." Occasionally a complete elaborate syntactic form, considerably beyond the child's current linguistic level, appears spontaneously, as when at age 2 years 9 months, Alister asked his Dad who had returned from a fishing trip, "Did you catch anything last night?" Judging by his question forms used for some time after, this question was probably learned and remembered in its entirety.

Little children delight in imitating their older brothers and sisters, their words as well as their actions. In some cases the older child may adopt the simpler language forms of the younger one, possibly to ensure that the game continues. Here is a bedtime routine of a 4-year-old boy and his 2-year-old brother, Martin.

Sit up, Martin	No sit up.
My library book.	My lib'y book.
Time to sit up.	Time to sit up.
Time to lie down.	Time to lie down.
Leave door open.	Leave door open.
Stand up.	Lie down.
Sit up.	Lie down.

etc.

Sometimes, nonsense words are introduced into such vocal and verbal play and may be used by the older child to evoke laughter or tears from the younger one.

New expressions are frequently invented by analogy as in "Hang down my coat" (cf. "Hang up my coat"). He may say "nothingwhere" for "nowhere," "somethingbody" for "somebody" and "nothingbody" for "nobody." Sometimes two expressions with similar meanings are fused to make one, as in "I don't fond of it," used by Alister at 2 years 6 months, which appears to be a cross between "I don't like it." and "I'm not fond of it." Adults are not exempt from such errors, "irregardless" being used instead of either "regardless" or "irrespective," for example. Should such a word be used by large numbers of people, it may become accepted as part of the language. Colloquial and idiomatic expressions are created by this process. Adults, as well as children, are prone to imitate their peers.

Talking in Sentences

Few adults attempting to learn a language attack the problem with the singlemindedness and persistence of the young child. He talks all day, either to others or to himself, commenting on what he is seeing or doing. As he listens and talks, he figures out many linguistic rules such as how to modify verbs when talking about what happened as compared with what is actually happening. At the single word stage he will simply use the word "see," later "see doggy" and "Me see doggy." He then learns a new vocabulary item, "saw," and uses that appropriately—"I saw a dog." Later, he becomes aware of the pattern of contrasts as in kick, kicked; play, played; jump, jumped, etc. and he then "corrects" his error, thus "I see-ed the dog." This new verb form may prove to be quite resistant to parental change, since it is based on a rule which overrides imitation. In another case, the child may find it hard to determine which word it is that requires the special ending. This is illustrated by the variants "That one waked up" and "He wake uped," which may co-exist for a while.

At times, conversation with the language-learning child seems to take on the form of an interrogation. He questions continually, sometimes asking for information, sometimes apparently verifying how one describes something verbally. From the relatively passive role of the listener in a storytelling situation, he becomes more directive. He asks, "What that boy doing?" "He going on bicycle?" "Where he is going?" "Why you do that?"

Unlike many adult language learners, the young child is not afraid to try out complicated constructions which he hasn't quite mastered. For example, at 2 years 5 months, Alister said to one of his friends who was running on the street, "No, no, my mummy said, not could running, no could not running."

By the time he is 3 or 4 years old, the young child has mastered the use of a range of question forms and negatives, including the extremely complicated rules relating to auxiliary verbs. Although he clearly cannot learn through imitation in its strict sense, he does depend on the presence of models. Adults and older children talk to him, and he responds. He questions and they respond. Learning from this continuing verbal interaction, the child's language conforms closer and closer to the language he hears spoken around him.

Summary of Factors Relating to the Rate of Language Acquisition

Why is it that some children speak much earlier and much more clearly than others, even those who are in the same family? Do certain children have a special flair for language, as others do for music or art, or is it more related to quantity and quality of parental input? Although we do not have adequate answers to these questions, we know that some of the prerequisite conditions for learning spoken language skills relate mainly to the child, while others relate to what people in his environment provide for him. The child must have adequate sensory mechanisms for speech reception and an intact central nervous system. From his environment he must derive security, stimulation, and reinforcement. There must be a warm, consistent, affectionate relationship with those who look after him, and pleasurable routines that establish and maintain his well-being. He must have a wide range of interesting activities and experiences, and he must be exposed to an abundance of normal speech and language patterns that are clearly related to the ongoing situation. He must be encouraged to listen and to imitate and be reinforced for babbling, for vocal communication, and for his first attempts at talking. He must experience success in establishing vocal and verbal communication.

Most hearing-impaired children can learn to understand and use fluent spoken language. By means of hearing aids, the use of vision and touch, and the provision of special training, most can learn to compensate for their hearing problem and develop adequate sensory mechanisms for speech reception. For most hearing-impaired children the greatest barrier to verbal learning is not their sensory deficit, but what people in their environment fail to provide for them. In the next six chapters we shall present basic information relating to the sound patterns of language, hearing, hearing aids, and speech. We shall then return to the discussion of spoken language, verbal communication, and special training for children who are hearing-impaired.

ANNOTATED BIBLIOGRAPHY

Abrahamsen, A. A.   *Child Language: An Interdisciplinary Guide to Theory and Research.* Baltimore, Md.: University Park Press, 1977.
This book is a gold mine for the researcher and serious student of child language. The author has provided a generously annotated bibliography organized by topic: General Resources, Syntactic Development, Semantic Development, Beyond Grammar, and Phonology and Orthography. Literature from related disciplines such as linguistics, cognitive psychology, adult psycholinguistics, Piagetian theory, philosophy of language, and artificial intelligence are included. There are approximately 1,500 entries, dating from 1894 to 1977.

Brown, R.   *A First Language: The Early Stages.* Cambridge, Mass.: Harvard University Press, 1973.
Roger Brown deals at length with results of his own studies on Adam, Eve, and Sarah as they begin to acquire syntax. He extends his discussion

to include semantic and cognitive aspects of child language. For graduate students and researchers.

Dale, P. S.   *Language Development: Structure and Function* (2nd Ed.) New York: Holt, Rinehart and Winston, 1976 (paperback).

The second edition of this book provides an introductory, yet fairly extensive overview of the literature on child language. Headings include First Words, Early and Later Syntax with chapters on Theories of Syntactic and Semantic Development. Dale also includes a section on Sign Language, but is not content with a description. Like certain other psychologists and linguists, he does not hesitate to step outside his field of competence and pronounce on the education of hearing-impaired children. He denigrates the "oral" approach, claiming (p. 52) that born deaf people could never learn language through speechreading! He is apparently unaware of the many who have done so and who have subsequently graduated from regular universities. He is also seemingly unaware of the technology which can nowadays be harnessed to exploit residual hearing and which facilitates the normal progression of language acquisition he so ably describes.

Fromkin, V., and Rodman, R.   *An Introduction to Language.* New York: Holt, Rinehart and Winston, 1974 (paperback).

Written with a humorous twist and illustrated with cartoons, this is probably the most comprehensive and easily read introduction to such topics as phonetics, phonology, semantics, syntax, and brain-processing. Suitable for students, teachers, and parents. Exercises are included.

Lenneberg, E. H., and Lenneberg, E. (Eds.)   *Foundations of Language Development. Vol. 1.* New York: Academic Press, 1975.

A collection of general articles, treating biological, phonologic, syntactic, semantic, and cognitive aspects of language development. Of interest to teacher/clinicians and students.

Schiefelbusch, R. L., and Lloyd, L. L. (Eds.)   *Language Perspectives: Acquisition, Retardation and Intervention.* Baltimore, Md.: University Park Press, 1974.

Research on a number of important themes is reviewed and discussed by knowledgeable contributors. P. Morse and P. Eims each report on infant speech perception. The development of concepts underlying language is discussed by Eve Clark, I. M. Schlesinger, and M. Bowerman. D. and A. Morehead present a Piagetian view of thought and language. Paula Menyuk covers the stage from babbling to words, while Lois Bloom gives her views on talking, thinking, and understanding. The aforementioned chapters deal with language acquisition. The text is suitable for graduate students and teacher/clinicians.

4. Speech Sounds, Hearing, and the Acoustics of English

*H*umans are capable of producing an extremely large variety of speech sounds. The sounds used in any given language are just a selection drawn from the many possibilities. In English, all speech sounds are produced as air is expelled through the mouth or the nose. In other languages (e.g., French or Portuguese), some speech sounds require the expulsion of breath through both the mouth and the nose. Yet other languages include sucking or clicking sounds, none of which is present in English, but many of which can be heard as babies babble.

Classification of Speech Sounds

As with any variety of objects or materials, speech sounds can be sorted into relatively few classes according to certain features they have in common. Thus, speech sounds can be classified as either *vowels* or *consonants*. English vowels are produced when the vocal cords vibrate and the breath stream passes directly over the tongue and out through the mouth. Consonants are produced when the tongue or the lips interrupts or diverts the breath stream in some way. Consonants that are usually produced with vibration of the vocal cords are termed *voiced*. Those that are produced without vocal cord vibration are labeled as *unvoiced*, or *voiceless*. Examples of voiced consonants are [m], [b], and [v]. Unvoiced consonants include such sounds as [s], [f], and [p]. Both vowels and consonants can be divided into further subsets.

Vowels

When we produce the vowels in the words "who," "would," and "know," the tongue is highly arched toward the back of the mouth. Accordingly, such vowels are known as *high back vowels.* When the tongue is arched low toward the back of the mouth, as in the words "more," "of," and "art," *low back vowels* are formed. When the highest part of the tongue is in the center of the mouth, as in the words "must" and "learn," *central vowels* are produced. English also contains *low front vowels* as in the words "and" and "then" and *high front vowels* such as those in the words "take," "his," and "ease." The position of the tongue in the mouth contributes most to shaping the pattern of the vowels we hear, although the position of the lips and the extent to which the jaw is opened also influence the acoustic properties of vowels.

Consonants

Consonants are classified not only according to whether they are voiced or voiceless, but also according to the *manner* in which they are produced. Different manners of production are best illustrated by contrasting the following sounds: [b] a *plosive* or *stop;* [w] a *semi-vowel;* [l] a *liquid;* [m] a *nasal;* [s] a *fricative;* and [tʃ] as in *ch*ur*ch*, an *affricate.* Each of these manners of production gives rise to a particular type of sound pattern. The different sound patterns associated with each manner of production will be described later on.

Finally, consonants are described according to their *place* of production, that is, according to the point where the vocal tract is maximally constricted during production of the sound. Place can be simply described as front, mid, or back. The plosives [b], [d], and [g] illustrate sounds that are produced at these three points. More precise description of place of production is afforded by specifying the organs or parts of the vocal tract involved in forming the maximal constriction. These are the lips, the tongue, the teeth, the alveolar ridge (located just behind the upper teeth), the palate (the roof of the mouth), the velum (the soft or moving part of the palate), and the glottis (the space between the vocal cords). On such a basis, seven distinctions of place are usually made in English. These are illustrated by the following: [b] a *bilabial;* [f] a *labiodental;* [θ] as in *th*ink, a *linguadental;* [d] a *lingua-alveolar;* [ʃ] as in *sh*ow, a *linguapalatal;* [g] a *linguavelar;* and [h] a *glottal* sound. Later on, we shall indicate how the resonances of the vocal tract tend to vary systematically according to a consonant's place of production.

Phonemes and Their Transcription

American English contains 43 phonemes: 14 vowels, 5 diphthongs, and 24 consonants. Phonemes are classes of sounds that differentiate one word from any other. Therefore, /b/ and /p/ are recognized as different phonemes because they differentiate the words "bill" and "pill." It is important to recognize that several different speech sounds can be classed as one phoneme. Thus, the [h] sounds in 'hoe," "hay," and "he" are the same phoneme even though they differ acoustically (whisper these words and the difference will be clearly audible). Different sounds classed as the same phoneme are called *allophones*. Most people are unaware that they use different allophones in different words or that another speaker's range of allophones may differ from their own. This is because attention is usually focused upon what is being said rather than upon how the speaker says it.

In written English, a 26-letter alphabet is used to represent the 43 phonemes. Thus, in order to write our language, two or more letters of the alphabet often have to be employed to specify a single phoneme. This is, for example, the case with the vowel sound in the word "p*ie*ce," and with the consonant in the word "*sh*e."

To write English phonetically, one must have a system of transcription that provides a symbol for each of the 43 phonemes. The most widely used system of this type is the International Phonetic Alphabet (IPA). In this alphabet the vowel in "piece" is written /i/ and the consonant in "she" is written /ʃ/. Placing such symbols between slash marks indicates that they represent phonemes drawn from meaningful speech. Placing them in square brackets indicates that the symbols have no reference to linguistic meaning.

In addition to a symbol for each phoneme, the person who attempts to make an exact transcription has to use diacritic markers. These markers, or modifiers, specify what allophones or phonetic variations were employed by a speaker in pronouncing particular words. For example, the word "heat" can be said with the final consonant deliberately aspirated (released with a puff of air), and this would be written /hit⁺/. Alternatively, the final consonant might be unreleased and this would be written /hit⁻/. The

IPA symbols and diacritic markers allow a much more precise description of speech faults than any other system of transcription. It is therefore the most appropriate system to use in describing speech development in hearing-impaired children. The IPA symbols are not difficult to learn, because most of them correspond closely to the alphabet used to write English. These symbols and the few modifiers that will be used in this book are shown, together with key words, on page vi of this book. Table 4.A uses these symbols to summarize the classification of English consonants according to their manner, place, and voicing characteristics.

Hearing for Speech

The phonemes specified in the previous section sound quite different from each other to the normal-hearing listener. To many hearing-impaired listeners, however, certain of these phonemes, if they can be heard at all, may sound much the same. In the following pages we shall describe the basic mechanisms of hearing, the acoustic properties of speech sounds, and how hearing impairment can affect auditory speech reception. Such information is essential for understanding the process of aural habilitation, which includes the selection and fitting of hearing aids, the use of residual audition, and the development of spoken language as a means of communication.

Speech sounds vary in several ways. They range from high to low, loud to quiet, and long to short. The identification of speech sounds through audition therefore requires that the listener be able to detect and discriminate changes in frequency (high-low), intensity (loud-quiet), and duration (long-short). These terms are used by scientists in a very specific way, as explained below. There are many sounds that are simply so quiet that no human can hear them, for they lie below the threshold of human hearing, beyond the limits of our auditory sensitivity. Some sounds are so high or so quiet that they cannot be detected by the human ear but can be heard by certain animals. Dogs, for example, can hear a whistle that is too high to be detected by the human ear.

Auditory Sensitivity

Tests to measure the threshold of hearing are carried out by the use of an audiometer. An audiometer is an instrument that produces tones of a given frequency at various levels of intensity. Before going further, let us examine what the words *frequency* and *intensity* mean and how they are measured.

Frequency

Frequency is measured in Hertz (Hz), the unit describing the number of vibrations per second giving rise to the sound. Thus, to create a sound of 125 Hz, a bee would beat its wings 125 times each second. To create a sound of 250 Hz, it would have to move its wings twice as fast. Most people can sing a 250 Hz note, which is about middle C (C_4) on the piano. For a woman it would be a low note, but for a man it would be quite high (the reason for this is explained later in this chapter). It is useful to relate the frequency scale on the audiogram to C on the piano. The octave above middle C (C_5) is about 500 Hz, the octave above that (C_6) is about 1000 Hz. The third octave above middle C (C_7) is about 2000 Hz. Top C on a full-size piano (C_8) is about 4000 Hz. Normal listeners can hear sounds from about 30 to 30,000 Hz. As one ages, sensitivity to high sounds tends to decrease substantially. Speech sounds occur over the whole range of frequency encompassed by the audiogram, from under 100 Hz to over 8000 Hz. Sounds below 125 Hz are more important in music than in speech. Indeed, it is not uncommon for people who have a high-frequency hearing loss to enjoy music even though they cannot hear speech very well.

When one hears a sound of a particular frequency, one thinks of it as having a certain pitch. The frequency of a sound is a physical reality; its pitch is our subjective judgment of its frequency. That frequency and pitch are not the same is illustrated by a condition known as *diplacusis*. A person with this condition, asked to listen to a tone of a certain frequency, would hear a higher pitched sound in one ear than in the other. Diplacusis may accompany some types of hearing impairment.

Intensity

Intensity is measured in decibels (dB). Zero dB on the audiogram is the average threshold of hearing for young, normal listeners. A wind gently moving the leaves of a tree would cause sound at about a 20 dB level. Whispered speech at a couple of yards would be at about a 40 dB level. At the same distance, average speech levels would be around 60 dB and a shout, around

TABLE 4.A

Consonants classified according to manner of production, place of production, and voicing.

		Bilabial	Labiodental	Linguadental	Alveolar	Palatal	Velar	Glottal
Plosives/Stops	Unvoiced	p			t		k	
	Voiced	b			d		g	
Fricatives	Unvoiced		f	θ	s	ʃ		h
	Voiced		v	ð	z	ʒ		
Nasals	Voiced	m			n		ŋ	
Semivowels	Voiced	w				j		
Liquids	Voiced				l, r			
Affricates	Unvoiced					tʃ		
	Voiced					dʒ		

(From *Speech and the Hearing-Impaired Child: Theory and Practice*, p. 259, © Alexander Graham Bell Association for the Deaf)

80 dB. A chain saw a few yards away would create noise levels of 100 dB or more. Exposure to continuous noise at levels above 100 dB for more than very brief periods could damage the auditory system and cause permanent hearing loss. The dB scale is logarithmic. Hence, sound at 100 dB is not twice as intense as sound at 50 dB, but several thousand times as intense. Doubling the intensity of a sound adds but 3 dB, and halving the intensity reduces its level by the same amount. Speaking to somebody from one yard away will result in levels that are about 6 dB greater than speaking with the same effort from a distance of two yards. The intensity of speech is raised by about 6 dB every time distance is halved. This is partly why speaking closer to a hearing-impaired child is more effective than raising one's voice level or increasing the amount of amplification provided by the hearing aid.

Intensity and loudness are related, but not identical, terms. Intensity is the quantity of sound that can actually be measured. Loudness is a perceptual judgment of the sound's magnitude. For example, should a sound of a certain intensity be presented to two different people, or two different ears of the same person, it will not sound equally loud if one of the people or one of the ears is hearing impaired. For normal listeners, loudness and intensity increase at much the same rate. However, some hearing-impaired listeners find that a very slight increase in the intensity of a sound results in a very large increase in its loudness. This phenomenon is known as *recruitment*.

Pure Tone Testing

A pure tone test is the most common measure of hearing. Its purpose is to determine the minimum level of intensity that a person requires in order to experience a sensation of sound. Typically, the person being tested wears headphones through which the tones are delivered. On hearing a tone, the person signals to the tester that the tone is audible. The tester then presents the same tone again at lower and lower intensity levels. The level at which the tone is barely audible (can be heard on about 50 percent of the presentations) is then recorded as the person's threshold. The same procedure is repeated for tones of different frequency. The various threshold levels obtained are usually plotted on a chart. This chart, known as an audiogram, is a graph of frequency versus intensity. An audiogram is shown as Figure 4.1.

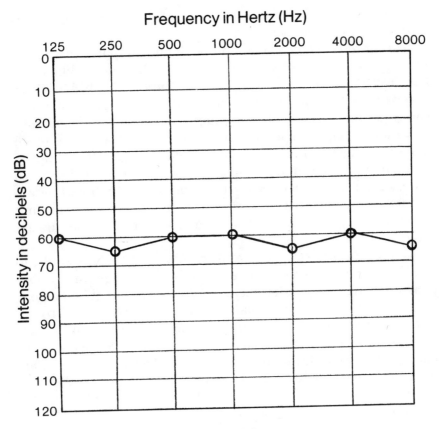

Figure 4.1

An audiogram depicting threshold levels for the right ear (circles). Normal hearing is 0 dB.

The audiogram depicted as Figure 4.1 shows a series of circles joined by a line about halfway down the chart. These circles represent the threshold levels obtained in testing the right ear of a person with impaired hearing. From this audiogram one can be quite sure that, without a hearing aid, the person would be unable to hear the rustle of leaves in the wind (20 dB), but would be able to detect some of the sounds of speech (60 dB). The audiogram, being based on the detection of simple (pure) tones, does not indicate how well (or poorly) the person tested is able to discriminate one sound from another, identify complex sounds, or comprehend amplified speech. The audiogram of a person with normal hearing would be at or near the top of the chart, at audiometric zero for all frequencies.

Hearing tests can be carried out without using headphones. If the purpose of the test is to determine whether the middle ear is defective, then the tones can be presented through a vibrator placed on the bone just behind the ear. If one wishes to test a baby who is too small to wear headphones, then special stimuli can be delivered through a speaker. If one wants to know how much amplification a hearing aid provides, then aided thresholds can be approximately determined while the hearing aid is being worn (see Chapter 7). Under most circumstances, tests should be administered in an environment where there is no background noise, and audiometry usually is carried out in a soundproof room.

To test a person's capacity to discriminate between sounds, to identify words, or to comprehend spoken language, more complex tests have to be undertaken. The audiogram is at best a poor guide as to how well a particular child will be able to learn through hearing. Children with normal thresholds of hearing rarely have difficulties in processing spoken language. However, hearing-impaired children with identical audiograms frequently have quite different capacities for use of their residual audition. We shall discuss the measurement and use of hearing more fully in Chapters 5, 6, and 7.

The Ear and Hearing

Once the presence of hearing impairment has been established, the next step is to determine what part of the child's auditory system is not functioning properly. In order to understand the tests that are used for this purpose, the reader must have at least an elementary knowledge of the ear. The essential details are depicted in Figure 4.2, which is a diagram (not drawn to scale) showing the major components of the auditory system.

Air Conduction

Sounds arrive at the ear as variations in air pressure. These variations travel, via the ear canal, to the ear drum, which moves in response to changes in air pressure. In turn, the movements of the ear drum cause corresponding motion across the chain of three small bones (the ossicular chain) that bridges the gap (the

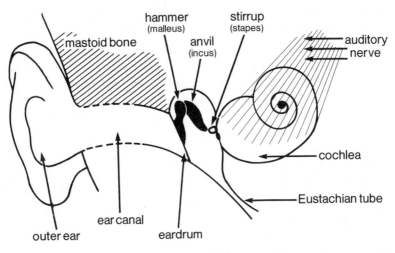

Figure 4.2

A diagram showing the main components of the ear. The outer ear and the middle ear (the part containing the three small bones—the ossicular chain) conduct sound to the inner ear (the cochlea). Faults in the outer or middle ear give rise to conductive loss. Faults in the cochlear or auditory nerve cause sensorineural loss.

middle ear cleft) between the ear drum and the cochlea—the organ in which the sensory nerve fibers are enclosed. The cochlea (sometimes called the inner ear) is a shell-like, spiral structure containing fluid. Vibration of the bones in the middle ear creates waves in this fluid, waves that stimulate the sensory fibers from which electrical (nerve) impulses travel to the brain. Low-frequency sounds create slow waves in the cochlear fluid which activate the nerve fibers farthest from the middle ear. High-frequency sounds create rapid waves that activate only those close to where the middle ear bones are connected to the cochlea. In some types of hearing impairment, fibers that normally detect high-frequency sounds are partly or wholly destroyed, while other fibers remain intact. This condition, which is not uncommon, results in high-tone hearing loss.

The above description of the ear and its functions indicates that the ear consists of two groups of components. One group—the ear canal and the middle ear structures—serves to conduct sound to the cochlea. Hearing impairment due to faults affecting these components is termed *conductive loss.* Such faults may be amenable to medical or surgical treatment. The other group—the sensory fibers and the auditory nerve—serve to create and transfer the resulting electrical impulses to the brain. Hearing impairment caused by faults in these structures is called *sensorineural loss.* Such faults permanently affect hearing, and nothing can be done to cure them.

Bone Conduction

If there is an impairment in the conductive components, such as wax blocking the ear canal, a perforation of the ear drum, or infection in the middle ear, then the intensity of vibrations reaching the inner ear will be reduced. To determine whether an impairment is conductive and whether the inner ear is normal, the audiologist can use impedance audiometry (see Chapter 5) or present sounds through a vibrator placed on the skull. The bones of the skull will then convey these vibrations directly to the cochlea. This phenomenon is known as *bone conduction.* Since the usual conductive mechanisms of the ear are thus by-passed, the patient with an impairment of these mechanisms will hear as well as a normal-hearing person under these conditions if the sensorineural mechanisms are intact. If normal responses are obtained through bone conduction, it follows that the impairment is not sensorineural and must therefore be conductive. On the other hand, if a person does not hear normally through bone conduction, it can be concluded that the hearing impairment is either partly or wholly of sensorineural origin. In order to test each ear independently through bone conduction, a noise has to be introduced into the ear not being tested so that vibrations conveyed to it through the skull are masked (covered up by the noise).

The otologist can often reach many of the same conclusions relating to conductive impairment as the audiologist. He may do this partly by examining the ear with an otoscope. Through this instrument he can see whether wax is blocking the ear, see if the ear drum is perforated, and detect the presence of middle ear abnormalities which lead to discoloration of the ear drum or pressure upon it. If he uses a pneumatic otoscope, i.e., an otoscope with a small rubber bulb connected to it, he can vary the air pressure in the ear canal by squeezing the bulb and thus determine whether the ear drum moves normally. If it does not, then he will usually be able to tell whether this is due to malfunction of the Eustachian tube (which allows the air pressure in the middle ear to become equalized with the air pressure in the ear canal), to fluid in the middle ear, to problems with the bones that form the ossicular chain, or some other difficulty. The otologist may also choose to find approximate thresholds or carry out bone conduction tests using tuning forks.

Once conclusions on the nature of a hearing impairment have been reached through audiologic and otologic assessment, treatment can be planned. If the hearing impairment is conductive, then it may be amenable to medical or surgical treatment. If it is sensorineural, it is permanent. It cannot be cured. The only form of treatment that can help the person with sensorineural loss is (re)habilitation. Some, if not all, speech sounds may be audible to such a person if they are appropriately amplified. What sounds will be audible in a given case can be fairly accurately deduced from a knowledge of two things: the person's audiogram and the acoustic properties of speech sounds.

The Acoustic Properties of Speech Sounds

An adequate breath stream is essential to the production of speech. When the vocal cords are brought together, the breath stream first pushes them apart and then acts, together with muscular tension, to close them. The vibration thus produced is the source of all voiced sounds. The rate at which the vocal cords vibrate (open and close) depends on their length, mass, and tension. The pitch of voice is determined by the rate at which the vocal cords vibrate. Since the vocal cords of adult males tend to have greater length and mass and thus tend to vibrate more slowly than those of adult females, male voices tend to be lower than females'. For the same reasons, female voices tend to be lower than those of young children. Within limits, the length, mass, and tension of the vocal cords can be changed through action of the laryngeal muscles; hence speakers can vary their intonation patterns through control of these muscles.

As the vocal cords open and close, a train of pulses, rich in harmonics, is created. If the vocal cords vibrate 100 times a second, then a fundamental pitch of 100 Hz is produced, and a larger series of harmonics is created at exact multiples of the fundamental pitch (200 Hz, 300 Hz, 400 Hz, etc.). If the vocal cords vibrate 200 times a second, then the fundamental pitch is

200 Hz, and harmonics occur at 400 Hz, 600 Hz, 800 Hz, and so on. The harmonics present in all voiced sounds are visible as horizontal bars in the spectrogram of the vowel [a] and the consonant [m] presented as Figure 4.3. The horizontal axis of a spectrogram represents time in seconds, and the vertical axis represents frequency in Hz. By counting the horizontal bars (harmonics) below 1000 Hz, the reader can deduce the approximate fundamental pitch of the speaker's voice. In Figure 4.3, there are 12 bars below 1000 Hz; hence one can deduce that the voice fundamental of the speaker was about 83 Hz (1000/12 = 83).

While the source of all voiced sounds is the larynx, specifically the vocal cords, the source of unvoiced sounds varies according to the point in the vocal tract at which turbulence is created. In whispered speech, the source of the sound is still the larynx. The

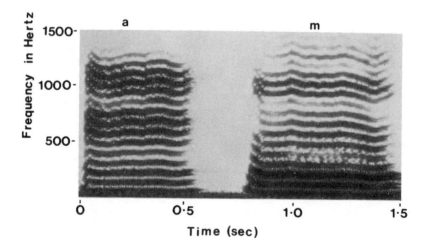

Figure 4.3

A narrow-band spectrogram of the vowel [a] and the consonant [m] spoken by a male with a deep bass voice. The horizontal lines show the harmonics present in his voice. The darker harmonics are those that are resonated in the oral cavity. These are the formants. In [a] the first formant is just above 600 Hz and the second, around 1000 Hz. In [m] the first formant is well below 500 Hz and the second, around 1000 Hz (see text).

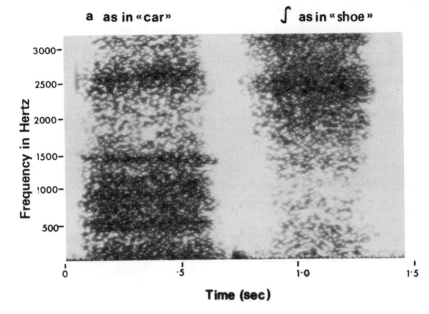

a as in «car»   **ʃ as in «shoe»**

Figure 4.4

A narrow-band spectrogram of the vowel [a], produced as a whisper. Note that there are no harmonics (no horizontal bars) but that the formants (resonances) are found in the same frequency regions as when the sound is voiced (see Figure 4.3). Also note that the [ʃ] similarly has no harmonics, since it is an unvoiced sound, and that most of the energy of the [ʃ], the darker marking, falls in the frequency range above 2000 Hz.

breath stream, driven through a partly open glottis, creates the sound we hear as a whisper by scattering the molecules of air in a random (aperiodic) manner. In unvoiced consonants, such as [ʃ] or [s], the turbulence is created by driving the breath stream through the aperture between the tongue and the palate or alveolar ridge and over the surfaces of the teeth. The random nature of such turbulence can be seen through examination of the spectrogram of the whispered vowel [a] and the consonant [ʃ] presented in Figure 4.4. Unlike the sounds depicted by the spectrogram shown as Figure 4.3, these unvoiced sounds contain no harmonics. The energy, instead of being concentrated in a series of horizontal bars, is scattered randomly throughout the frequency range of these sounds.

The periodic vibrations of the vocal cords in voiced sounds and the aperiodic turbulence in unvoiced sounds give speech its energy. But it is the shape and motion of the vocal tract that give phonemes their main characteristics. The vocal tract serves as a filter which selectively allows some sounds to be resonated while other sounds are damped to the point of inaudibility. Because the tongue, jaw, and lips can assume a variety of positions, the shape of the vocal tract can be modified to create a variety of sounds. In the following paragraphs, we shall show how the resonance/filter effects described above give rise to the particular vowels and consonants we use in English.

Vowels

When the tongue is raised high toward the back of the mouth, the lips are rounded, and the jaw is slightly open, part of the vocal tract assumes a shape similar to that of a bottle with a narrow neck. If one blows across the neck of such a bottle so that the air molecules inside are set into vibration, then an [u]-like sound (as in the word "who") is produced. Similarly, the vowel [u] will result when we use a voice or whisper to energize the air molecules in the vocal tract with the tongue, lips, and jaw in such positions. The resonances, or *formants,* thus generated will be low-frequency sounds, one (the first formant or F_1) centered around 300 Hz and the other (the second formant or F_2) around 800 Hz. There will be little or no high-frequency energy present in such a vowel, because the upper harmonics (if voiced) and the high-pitched turbulence (if whispered) cannot resonate in such a vocal tract configuration.

As the highest point of the arch created by the tongue moves forward in the mouth, the second formant (F_2) of the vowel produced will rise in frequency. The effect is akin to blowing across the neck of a bottle after more and more water has been added. The higher the water level in the bottle, the higher will be the note produced. When the highest point of the tongue is in the center of the mouth (as in the vowel [a]), the center frequency of F_2 will be just over 1000 Hz. When the highest point of the tongue is very

Figure 4.5 (opposite): *A diagram showing the approximate frequency range of the first and second formants of the English vowels as spoken by adult males. If hearing impairment renders sound above 1000 Hz inaudible, then some back and front vowels will sound similar and may be confused.*

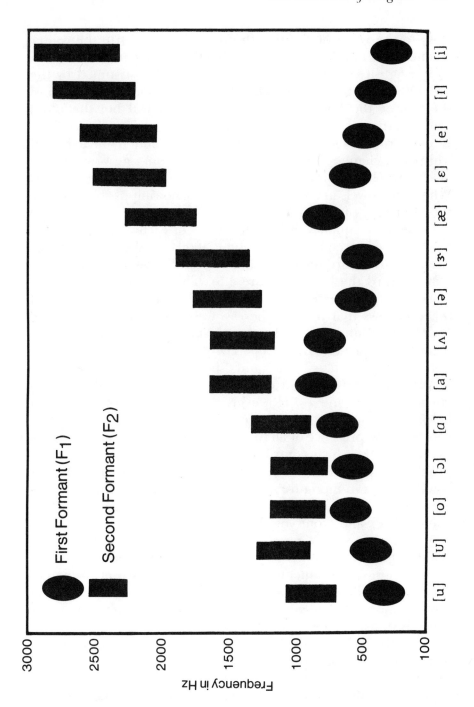

close to the front of the mouth (as in the vowel [i]), the center frequency of F_2 will be well over 2000 Hz. The rise in frequency of F_2 in English vowels is assisted by the positions assumed by the lips. Other things being equal, the larger the opening of the lips, the higher the frequency of the formants will be; the more rounded the lips, the lower the frequency of the formants will be. If one produces the three vowels [u], [a], and [i] in a forced whisper, a change in the frequency of F_2 from one vowel to the next can be heard quite clearly as a change in pitch of the whisper. When the vowels are voiced it is hard, if not impossible, to hear the frequency of formants.

While the frequency of F_2 is different for each vowel, that of F_1 tends to rise in frequency from about 300 Hz as the tongue moves from the [u] toward the [a]. F_1 then falls as the tongue continues to move toward the [i] (see Figure 4.5). Thus F_1 for several vowel pairs is quite similar — for example, [u] and [i], [ʊ] and [ɪ], [ɔ] and [ɛ]. It follows that if F_2 of these vowels cannot be heard, these vowel pairs sound quite alike. As a result, severe hearing impairment for frequencies over 1,000 Hz often causes auditory confusion of words such as "shoe" and "she."

All vowels also have third formants (F_3) that are higher in frequency than F_1 and F_2. However, they play little or no role in helping the listener to differentiate between one vowel and another. The presence of all formants gives speech a natural quality, but it is F_2 which contributes most to intelligibility. The approximate center frequencies of the first two formants of each vowel are shown in Figure 4.5. Note how F_2 rises as the tongue is advanced in the mouth, and note the similarities in F_1 for certain pairs of back and front vowels.

Diphthongs

Diphthongs are phonemes that glide from one vowel position to another. The diphthong [aɪ], for example, begins with the vowel [a] and ends with the vowel [ɪ]. It is present in the word "kite," which is transcribed in phonetics as /kaɪt/. If this word were produced with either one of these vowels alone, it would be heard as /kat/ — the Bostonian pronunciation of "cart," or as /kɪt/ — as in the word "kit." To determine the approximate frequencies of the glides in the diphthongs of English, one may join the first formants and then the second formants of the two vowels which form the sound, e.g. [aɪ], [ɔɪ] or [eɪ]. Joining F_1 of [a] and [ɪ], for example, would yield a glide from just under 1000 Hz to just over 300 Hz; joining F₂ of these vowels would yield a glide in the opposite direction, from just over 1000 Hz to just under 3000 Hz. The formant glides in the diphthongs [aɪ], [ɔɪ], and [aʊ] are shown in Figure 4.6.

Consonants

Consonants rarely occur in isolation during running speech. They usually serve to release or arrest vowels and other consonants. Depending on which vowel or consonant they release or arrest, their acoustic properties change. For example, /k/ in the word "key" is much higher in frequency than /k/ in the word "cool." The /k/ in "clown" is neither as high as one, nor as low as the other. These differences can be heard most clearly in whispered speech. Because consonants interact systematically with adjacent sounds, the acoustic transitions that result as the speech organs move from one sound to the next help to identify which consonant was spoken. These changing acoustic patterns are con-

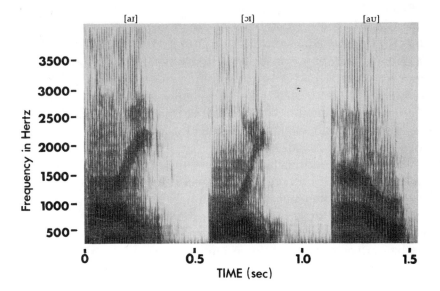

Figure 4.6

A broad-band spectrogram of the three diphthongs [aɪ], [ɔɪ] and [aʊ] showing how the formants change continuously as the tongue glides from the initial to the final vowel position.

sidered as offering *variant cues.* Of course, each consonant also has characteristic acoustic properties that differentiate it from others, regardless of context. These properties are considered as offering *invariant cues.*

Manner of consonant production is signaled principally by invariant acoustic cues. *Plosives* are characterized by a brief silence over most of the speech frequency range, lasting about 30–50 milliseconds (msec) prior to a burst of noise. The silence and subsequent noise burst are the acoustic results of stopping the breath flow with the lips, as in [p], or with the tongue, as in [t] or [k], and then suddenly releasing the pressure that has been built up. *Semivowels* and *liquids* are characterized by rapidly changing energy in the low- to mid-frequency range. Invariant cues for *nasals* include a low-frequency murmur (about 250–300 Hz) and a series of antiresonances just above the formants. *Fricatives* are characterized simply by a smooth, high-frequency hiss, an aperiodic sound created by the turbulence of the breath stream. *Affricates* combine some of the properties of both stops and fricatives in that a high-frequency hiss is preceded by the silent interval imposed by closing the vocal tract with the tongue.

Place of consonant production is signaled largely by variant cues. Sounds made at the front of the mouth, such as [p], [b], [m], and [f], produce F_2 transitions that start under 1000 Hz and rise in frequency. Alveolar consonants such as [t], [d], [n], and [s] are associated with F_2 transitions that tend to start in the mid-frequency range (about 1800 Hz) and then fall or rise in frequency depending on vowel contexts. Consonants made at the back of the mouth, such as [g] and [k], tend to produce F_2 transitions that fall in frequency.

Voicing distinctions among consonants are signaled by both invariant and variant cues. The invariant acoustic cue to voicing is, of course, the presence of a fundamental pitch and a range of harmonics generated by vibration of the vocal cords. Perception of the voiced-voiceless distinction can, however, occur solely on the basis of variant cues. Such cues are provided by the relative durations of the vowel and consonant in a syllable. Even if the final consonant is made without vocal cord vibration, it will be perceived as voiced if it is significantly shorter than the preceding phoneme. Thus, the words "hiss" and "his" can be differentiated in whispered speech because "his" normally has a long vowel and a short fricative and "hiss" usually has a short vowel and a long fricative.

Conversational Speech

In conversational speech, the phonemes discussed above do not follow each other like letters on a printed page. Nor are words produced as separate entities. Speech is usually produced as a stream of coarticulated sounds, each influenced by those that precede or follow it. Yet native speakers and listeners are able to segment this stream into words and, if necessary, into phonetic units. Segmentation skills are achieved through attending to patterns of rhythm, stress, and intonation that mark the boundaries

where are you going?

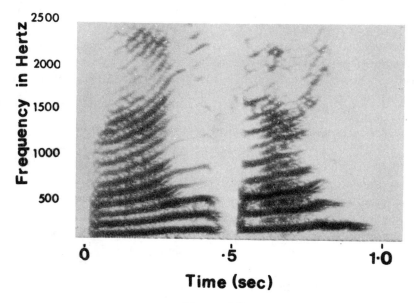

Figure 4.7
A narrow-band spectrogram of the question "Where are you going?" spoken by an adult male, which shows how all the harmonics rise as fundamental voice frequency (F_0) is increased. At the outset, F_0 is about 100 Hz, and at the end of the sentence, about 250 Hz, a rise of more than an octave.

of sentences, words, and syllables. These patterns, relative to phonetic segments, are slowly changing. For example, several words comprising many phonemic segments may be used to formulate a question which has but a single rising intonation pattern. Because such patterns extend over a number of phonetic segments, they are truly suprasegmental.

Some suprasegmental patterns—such as intonation and word stress—are carried by voicing, i.e., by vowels and voiced sounds involving vibration of the vocal cords. Intonation not only makes speech pleasant to listen to and points up word and sentence boundaries; it can also change the meaning of a word or a sentence. Stress, which includes changes in frequency, intensity, and duration of voicing, acts in a similar fashion. Fortunately, because most suprasegmental patterns are carried by the harmonics which are resonated in the F_1 of voiced sounds, they can be made audible even to children with hearing only for low-frequency speech sounds.

A spectrogram showing the intonation pattern of the sentence "Where are you going?" is shown in Figure 4.7. In this spectrogram the harmonics are seen to rise in frequency throughout the sentence. All the sounds in this sentence are voiced, hence the intonation pattern is continuous across all words except for the break in voicing which signals the plosive /g/ at the beginning of the last word.

Acoustic Patterns and Hearing Impairment

More detailed descriptions of the acoustic properties of English phonemes are available in Ling (1976) and other texts listed in the bibliography for this chapter. From the data presented above, however, it is possible to make certain statements that have important implications relating to auditory speech reception by hearing-impaired children who are suitably fitted with hearing aids.

First, all vowels have first formant (F_1) energy below 1000 Hz. Hence they should be audible to a child if his residual hearing extends to that frequency.

Second, since several vowel pairs have similar first formant (F_1) frequencies, confusions between them may occur if second formants (F_2) of these vowels are not also audible to the child. Positive identification of all vowels demands hearing up to at least 2500–3000 Hz.

Third, some consonants cannot be produced in isolation because both variant and invariant cues are only available when the consonant is used to release or arrest an adjacent sound.

Fourth, manner distinctions among consonants can be made by children who have hearing only for low-frequency speech sounds. This is because most are signaled by acoustic cues throughout the range of speech frequencies.

Fifth, place distinctions among consonants are signaled by acoustic cues that lie mainly in the frequency range 1,500–3,000 Hz. Children whose hearing for this frequency range is poor are therefore likely to have difficulty in hearing differences between sounds such as [p], [t], and [k].

Sixth, voicing distinctions among consonants are signaled both by the harmonics generated by vibration of the vocal cords and by the relative duration of adjacent sounds. Since both of these cues are present well under 1000 Hz, children with hearing only for low-frequency speech sounds should be able to differentiate voiced and unvoiced sounds if they are fitted with appropriate hearing aids.

ANNOTATED BIBLIOGRAPHY

Fry, D. B. (Ed.)   *Acoustic Phonetics.* New York and London: Cambridge University Press, 1976.
Described by the author as a course of basic readings in acoustic phonetics, this text is made up of more than 30 rather advanced-level articles culled from the literature published during this century. It includes papers that may be considered as among the most important in the field. It is highly recommended for teacher/clinicians working with hearing-impaired children, students who wish to do so, and parents with a scientific bent who can discuss the various topics covered with someone knowledgeable.

Ladefoged, P.   *A Course in Phonetics.* New York: Harcourt, Brace, Jovanovich, 1975.
A first-rate introductory text that covers the major aspects of phonetics clearly and systematically, this book is particularly useful to teacher/clinicians who want to brush up their phonetics and students who like to learn through painless reading. The author makes but few references to source material, which is a serious disadvantage for the reader who wishes to pursue certain topics in more detail.

Ling, D.   *Speech and the Hearing-Impaired Child: Theory and Practice.* Washington, D.C.: A.G. Bell Association for the Deaf, 1976.
The acoustic properties of speech and their relationships to various types and levels of hearing impairment are described. The application of phonetics in teaching speech production skills to hearing-impaired children is discussed throughout this text. Abundant references to original work in acoustic and articulatory phonetics are provided.

O'Connor, J. D.   *Phonetics.* Baltimore, Md.: Penguin Books, 1973.
This introductory treatment of various aspects of phonetics includes how speech sounds are produced, the acoustics of speech, how speech sounds are perceived by normal listeners, and the relationship between sounds and language. The text is easy to read and, as a paperback, inexpensive to purchase.

Singh, S., and Singh, K.   *Phonetics: Principles and Practices.* Baltimore, Md.: University Park Press. 1976.
An introductory text on phonetics with abundant illustrations. The most elementary treatment of the topic available. Pictures of lip and tongue positions are provided, some of which, unfortunately, appear to be exaggerated. Exercises (questions) to serve as a self-check on comprehension are included. Answers are given at the back of the book. The authors give no references to other publications.

Tiffany, W. R., and Carrell, J.   *Phonetics: Theory and Application.* New York: McGraw Hill, 1977.
A comprehensive treatment of phonetic science, this book is an extensive revision of a widely acclaimed classical text by the same authors (Carrell and Tiffany, 1960). Concepts are covered in depth, yet in a style that is suitable for readers who do not have extensive background. The book includes chapters that cover transcription, articulation, and acoustic phonetics. The dynamic nature of speech is stressed.

5.   Audiologic Assessment

Most children in whom some degree of deafness is suspected are examined by otologists (medical specialists concerned with ear problems) and tested by audiologists (clinicians who specialize in the science of hearing). In this chapter we shall describe the tests most frequently used in audiologic assessment, explain their purpose, and indicate how the results of such assessment are used in planning a child's medical or educational treatment. The reader will find that the material presented below extends the concepts introduced in Chapter 4.

In most cases, a child's hearing problems are first suspected by parents or other members of the child's family. Usually, the bases of such suspicions are the child's failure to respond to certain sounds, his lack of speech development, or both. In a small proportion of children, hearing impairment is suspected because one or more members of the family have a life-history of hearing difficulties.

Children with normal hearing usually startle to loud, unexpected sounds and cry as do other babies, from the first few days of life. They quiet to a soothing voice from a few weeks of age, move their eyes toward the source of a quiet sound from about 3 months of age, turn their heads in the direction of a quiet sound such as a whisper from about 6 months of age, and begin to show evidence of understanding a few words around their first birthday. Children who are hearing impaired from birth do not follow this course of development. In the early months, most babies coo and gurgle, even those with hearing impairment. Normal-hearing babies go on to babble strings of syllables from about 6 months of age, to acquire first words at about a year, and to use two words together by 18 months to 2 years. Children who are hearing impaired from birth tend to vocalize less frequently from about 6 months of age, and may become silent by 2 years of age. If they continue to vocalize, they usually produce patterns that are more typical of younger infants. At the same time, they respond readily to visual stimuli. Some 50 years ago, before audiologists, instruments, and procedures were available to test hearing, early childhood deafness was diagnosed solely on the basis of observations of different behaviors such as those described above. Even now, audiologists include such observations in their assessments, and rightly so.

There is considerable variability among children. Some children develop more quickly or slowly than suggested above. Others fail to respond to sound or develop speech normally, not because they have a hearing impairment, but because something else is amiss. Such children commonly include those who are autistic, severely mentally retarded, or brain damaged. Children with handicaps of this type may also be hearing impaired. Audiologic assessment of infants therefore demands a thorough knowledge of normal and deviant child development.

Hearing impairment can be caused by illness or accident at any time during childhood. If it occurs after speech and language have been acquired, the audiologist may be able to use word discrimination tests as part of the assessment. If it occurs before verbal skills have developed, then the tests and procedures used in the assessment will be similar to those employed with children who are hearing impaired from birth.

Behavioral Tests

There are three main types of behavioral tests: (1) those in which the child's responses to various sounds are simply observed; (2) those in which the child responds voluntarily each time he hears the test sound—by raising his hand, for example, or putting a peg in a pegboard; and (3) those in which the child's responses are rewarded and thus reinforced.

Tests of the first type have much in common with the observations made by parents, as discussed above. The major difference is that the sounds, or stimuli used by the audiologist to test the child are of known intensity, frequency, duration, and complexity.

They are presented in a controlled environment through calibrated equipment, and the responses of the child are noted and compared to those made by many other children.

Tests of the second type were described in Chapter 4. Tests of the third type require that something is done or made to happen, immediately following the stimuli, that will lead the child to respond again when the next stimulus is heard. For example, a window with attractive puppets may be made to light up if the child looks up immediately after a test sound is presented. Or, a television screen may be used to display a sequence of moving patterns; the child may be allowed to move an object or be given a token or a trinket. The type of reinforcement selected by the audiologist will depend upon the age and interests of the child.

In tests of all three types, a variety of stimuli can be used. Young babies respond more readily to complex sounds than to pure tones, to different sounds more readily than to the same sound repeated several times, and to sounds that are produced near to, rather than far away from, him. Whatever stimuli are used, the purpose of the test is to determine the child's threshold of detection for sounds, so that his hearing levels can be estimated relative to those of normal-hearing children.

Because very young children do not respond to sounds at their threshold of hearing, there is always a certain amount of educated guesswork in interpreting their responses to behavioral tests. Some very severely hearing-impaired children do not initially respond to sound at all; yet later tests show that they can hear some sounds at high-intensity levels.

Instrumental Tests

Instrumental tests are those in which involuntary responses to sound are automatically obtained and recorded, and all that is required of the child is that he submits to the test. Such tests are sometimes termed "objective tests." Since there is room for error in their administration and in the interpretation of results obtained, we consider the use of the term "objective" to be misleading. Several types of instrumental tests have been developed of which impedance audiometry, evoked response audiometry, and cochleography are the most frequently used. Instrumental tests that are less routinely employed (and will not be discussed below) include those that measure responses to sound through recording changes in heart rate and skin resistance. With the exception of impedance audiometry, instrumental tests are most often used with children when their behavioral responses cannot be readily obtained.

Impedance Audiometry

Impedance audiometry can be carried out with patients of all ages. The first impedance measure we shall describe is known as tympanometry. It determines how much sound is reflected from the ear drum as its tension is changed through the increase or decrease of air pressure in the ear canal. The principle is simple: If one were to throw a small object against a drapery that is hanging loosely, it would hit the drapery and fall. If one were to throw the same object against a drapery that is tightly stretched, it would bounce back into the room. The energy of sound is similarly absorbed by a flaccid ear drum and reflected by an ear drum that is tense. The ear drum is not usually under pressure, since air can normally enter the middle ear via the Eustachian tube. The normal ear therefore reflects relatively little sound energy. If the Eustachian tube is blocked, however, the air in the middle ear cleft will become absorbed by the surrounding tissue. Air pressure in the ear canal will become greater than that in the middle ear, and the ear drum will become abnormally tense. Such a problem may result from a cold. Under these conditions, the ear drum will reflect more than the normal amount of sound energy. This is why people who wear hearing aids often find that more feedback (acoustic howl) occurs when they have a cold.

To test impedance, the audiologist places a probe in the ear canal. Three channels run through the probe: One is used to deliver a tone to the ear, another leads to a microphone so that the quantity of sound reflected from the ear drum can be measured, and the third is connected to an air pressure system. The probe is seated so that air will not leak from the ear canal. Changes in the amount of sound reflected as air pressure is increased or decreased are automatically recorded on a chart. The resulting graph is called a tympanogram. From the shape of the tympanogram, the audiologist can judge whether there is a problem affecting the middle ear structures that could cause conductive hearing impairment and, if so, what type of problem it is likely to be. The test is particularly useful as an adjunct both to otoscopic evaluation by an otologist and to bone conduction audiometry.

The apparatus employed in tympanometry can also be used to measure the extent to which a reflex tightening of the ear drum occurs when sound of a particular intensity is presented. This reflex measure is sometimes helpful in demonstrating whether a person with sensorineural impairment has recruitment, i.e., hears sounds as very much louder than others when their intensity is actually increased very little (see Chapter 4). Such information helps in selecting hearing aids that will amplify speech to adequate levels but prevent uncomfortably loud sounds from reaching the ear. In certain cases, reflex audiometry can also be used to determine whether or not hearing levels in both ears are equal.

Evoked Response Audiometry
Evoked response audiometry is a procedure in which the electrical activity in various parts of the brain is measured as numerous acoustic stimuli (brief bursts of noise or tones) are presented. Such activity is detected through the use of electrodes pasted to the child's scalp. The output from these electrodes is then amplified and fed to a computer which averages the electrical signals it receives from the brain. Since responses to stimuli follow a systematic pattern, and the noise in the system is random, this process separates the response pattern from the noise. Patterns that are obtained can be displayed on a screen or automatically charted on paper. When clear patterns emerge, they provide evidence that the child's auditory system is capable of detecting the stimuli that were presented. Different parts of the pattern are associated with activity in different parts of the brain. Those parts of the pattern which have short latency (appear a few milliseconds after the stimulus is presented) originate in the brainstem and are termed brainstem evoked responses (BER). Those that originate at the cortex have longer latency and are termed the auditory evoked response (AER). They occur hundreds of milliseconds after the stimulus is presented. Both types of response are used in advanced clinical testing.

Cochleography
When sound arrives in the normal cochlea, the nerve fibers in the cochlea generate an electrical potential which has the same pattern as the stimulus. In this regard, the cochlea acts somewhat like a microphone, hence this electrical potential is called the *cochlear microphonic*. This activity in the cochlea triggers a pattern of

electrical impulses which travel along the auditory (eighth) nerve to the brain. These electrical impulses are called the *action potential*. The measurement of these particular electrical potentials is called *cochleography*. Cochleography can indicate whether hearing impairment is present and, if so, whether it is conductive, originates in the cochlea, or is due to eighth nerve dysfunction (see Chapter 4).

Both the cochlear microphonic and the action potential are very weak signals even when they are detected and recorded through an electrode placed in the most suitable location. The signals picked up by the electrode have to be amplified, therefore, and then processed by a computer in much the same way as the signals obtained in evoked response audiometry (see above). Because the signals received from the cochlea and the eighth nerve are extremely weak if they are recorded from an electrode placed on the surface of the skull or on the ear lobe, most workers place an electrode either on the ear drum or through the ear drum onto the cochlea. Such electrode placement demands that the child be placed under general anesthesia. The audiologist therefore has to work in collaboration with one or more physicians in order to carry out this test. Predictably, the procedure is far from routine in most clinics—even in those having the equipment.

Planning Treatment

The various tests described above are designed to establish whether or not hearing impairment is present and, if so, to define the type and extent of the problem. On the basis of knowledge derived from such tests, it is possible for members of a specialist team to decide upon the forms of treatment that are most appropriate for a child and to recommend such treatment to the child's parents.

Medical and/or surgical treatment is usually indicated if there is a conductive impairment. Most conductive problems are amenable to such intervention, although there are some occasions when surgical treatment is avoided on account of certain hazards. As an extreme example, imagine a child who has lost all hearing in one ear as a result of having had mumps and who has severe mixed (conductive and sensorineural) impairment in the other. Since all surgery is attended by a certain risk, however small, it might be considered more appropriate to provide such a child with extra amplification than to have him undergo surgery and possibly lose the hearing in this ear as a result. In such cases, so much depends on the exact nature of the problem and the degree of risk involved that generalizations would be of no value.

If hearing impairment is found to be of sensorineural origin, it is neither temporary nor amenable to medical or surgical treatment. The only thing that can help a child with sensorineural impairment is technical and educational help—(re)habilitation. This may take several forms, depending on the degree of hearing impairment and the child's age at its onset. Children with average hearing levels of 20 dB or less should be able to learn spoken language skills spontaneously and participate in family or school life without a hearing aid. If they are of school age, an advantageous position in class might be all that is required. Children with sensorineural impairment at levels averaging greater than 25 to 30 dB probably require hearing aids. Their parents usually need help in order to deal with (or better still avoid) the problems normally associated with such impairment, and both may need long-term assistance of a skilled teacher/therapist. Because this book is written for the benefit of such children, all other chapters relate to these needs.

Speech Tests of Hearing

In the preceding sections we have discussed tests employing noise or tonal stimuli designed to determine threshold of hearing. Speech sounds, words, and sentences can also be used as the stimuli in a variety of behavioral tests. Indeed, speech reception thresholds are commonly obtained from children with spoken language skills in order to check the validity of the tests described above. They are usually determined with *spondee words* (words with two equally stressed syllables such as "sidewalk" and "airplane"). Speech sounds are complex in nature; each sound covers a wide range of frequencies (see Chapter 4). Therefore they cannot be used—as can pure tones or calibrated noise—to determine precise thresholds of hearing. Because of this, speech tests of hearing are used in diagnostic audiology less frequently than in rehabilitative audiology. Their greatest contribution is the information they provide for two purposes: (1) selecting hearing aids, and (2) evaluating the effects of training the child to use his residual hearing. For these purposes, such tests include all four levels of speech reception: detection, discrimination, identification, and comprehension.

Terms relating to speech tests of hearing are often used inappropriately. Therefore the unwary reader may wrongly equate speech *reception* thresholds with speech *detection* thresholds. When the audiologist asks the listener to say which spondee is heard, he is using either a discrimination test (if the set from which the spondee is selected is known to the listener), or an identification test (if it is not). The scores obtained when a listener is asked to repeat words presented from a list of monosyllables are commonly referred to as *discrimination scores.* They are more frequently *word identification scores* since the listener is not usually told what words are likely to be presented. This is not a trivial matter. A discrimination task is much easier than an identification task, and therefore better scores are likely to be obtained on discrimination tests.

True discrimination tests are concerned with whether stimuli are the same or different. They often take the form AB, X, or ABC, X where A, B, and C are words that are known and X is the test word presented. Such tasks can also take the opposite form, namely X, ABC. Thus, showing a child a set of three pictures (ABC), naming them, and then asking him to point to one of the pictures (X) is a discrimination task. In the case of an AB, X set, the child has only two choices and can be right 50 percent of the time by chance. With sets of three, the chance level is one in three or 33.3 percent, and with sets of four, 25 percent. Hearing-impaired children often have to be taught the words before discrimination tests can be administered. The identification task demands that the child correctly repeats the test word on the basis of having identified the whole word pattern or a sufficient number of its elements. Because young or severely hearing-impaired children often have too little command of spoken language to say many words correctly, identification tests are seldom administered other than by persons who are concerned with educating the child to use residual hearing. We shall discuss speech tests of hearing as they relate to the selection of hearing aids in Chapter 6 and as they relate to the use of residual hearing in Chapter 7.

ANNOTATED BIBLIOGRAPHY

Davis, H., and Silverman, S. R. (Eds.)   *Hearing and Deafness.* 4th Ed. New York: Holt, Rinehart, and Winston, 1978.
A comprehensive text about hearing and deafness. It provides details on almost any aspect of audiology and hearing impairment that the reader is likely to need. Numerous authors contributed to the text, which is written in a style that is reasonably easy to read.

Katz, J. (Ed.)   *Handbook of Clinical Audiology.* Baltimore, Md.: Williams and Wilkins, 1972.
This very comprehensive handbook contains a few chapters relating to the audiologic assessment of children. It is a text written for professional workers by experts in each of the several aspects of the field. Each chapter contains numerous references.

Martin, F. N.   *Introduction to Audiology.* Englewood Cliffs, N.J.: Prentice-Hall, 1975.
Excellent introductory material on audiology. Each chapter begins with a statement on content and ends with a quiz. All chapters are well illustrated, and references to other books and articles are provided for each topic covered.

Northern, J. L., and Downs, M. P.   *Hearing in Children.* Baltimore, Md.: Williams and Wilkins, 1974.
This text offers the most exhaustive treatment of hearing impairment in children that is currently available. The authors present facts and references on causation, development of auditory behavior, testing procedures, and hearing aids. In Chapter 8, they unfortunately allow their enthusiasm for sign language to obscure both facts and judgment. The authors clearly have inadequate expertise in habilitation and education of hearing-impaired children. This should not deter the reader, however, for the authors' points of view are frequently encountered and should be understood. Their credibility and competencies in diagnostic aspects of audiology are unquestioned; the book is strongly recommended both as a text and as an excellent source of references.

6. Hearing Aids

*H*earing aids are the most important tool available to hearing-impaired children. Since few such children are totally deaf, most can benefit from their use, and most can hear better with two aids than with one. Because hearing impairment varies from one child to another, the most appropriate personal hearing aids for any given child must be selected from the large range of instruments that are available. There are no hearing aids that can be considered as "best" for all children, but there are usually particular aids that suit a given child's needs better than others.

Individual hearing aids are made in a variety of shapes and sizes. They may be carried on the body, housed in the frames of eyeglasses, worn over the ear, or fitted directly into the ear canal. A few deliver amplified sound to the ear through a vibrator placed firmly against the mastoid bone. Various types of hearing aids in current use are shown in Figure 6.1. Body-worn instruments are equipped with cords and receivers that carry and deliver the amplified signals from the hearing aid to the ear. Amplified sound is directed into the ear canal through an earmold. To ensure that earmolds fit comfortably and work effectively, they are cast in plastic from an impression taken of the entrance to the ear canal and the surrounding structures. Hearing aids that are fitted directly into the ear canal are bonded to the earmold.

A variety of special-purpose hearing aids are also used by hearing-impaired children at home, in clinics, or in school. Such special-purpose aids include radio aids, amplifying units that stand on, or are fixed to, a table and deliver sound through head-

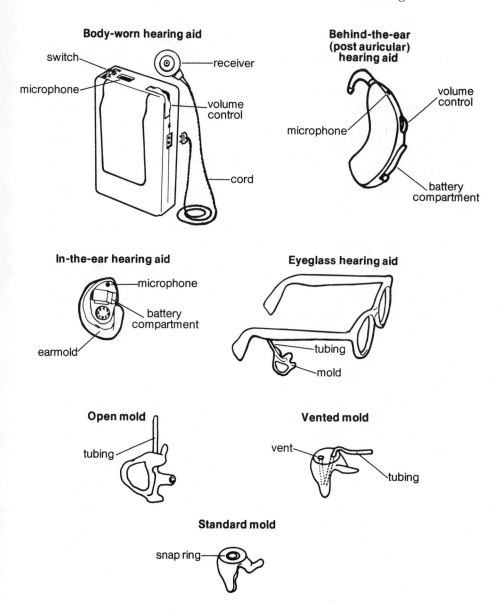

Body-worn hearing aid

switch

microphone

receiver

volume control

cord

Behind-the-ear (post auricular) hearing aid

volume control

microphone

battery compartment

In-the-ear hearing aid

microphone

battery compartment

earmold

Eyeglass hearing aid

tubing

mold

Open mold

tubing

Vented mold

vent

tubing

Standard mold

snap ring

Figure 6.1

Diagrams of different types of hearing aids and earmolds. Most manufacturers make a variety of models of each type of hearing aid. Earmolds are usually custom fitted, and many variations of the three basic forms depicted above can be produced from an impression of an individual's ear.

phones (hard-wire systems), and loop induction systems. These special-purpose aids will be described and discussed in the next chapter.

There are three main parts to every hearing aid: the microphone, which detects the sound and converts it into electrical energy; the amplifier, which increases the intensity of the signal received; and the receiver, which converts the electrical energy back into sound. The quality of these components is constantly being improved, and each part has become increasingly miniaturized as technology has advanced. Hearing aids differ partly because the microphones, amplifiers, and receivers used in hearing aids are not necessarily of the same type or quality, and partly because these components are not put together in the same way. The power needed to drive personal hearing aids is provided by a small battery (cell). The quantity and quality of amplification a hearing aid produces can be influenced by the strength of the cell. Some hearing aids require more electrical current to operate than others and will drain the cells more quickly and are thus less economical to run.

The selection of the most appropriate instruments for a child is not a simple matter. First, the electroacoustic and control features most suitable to him must be determined. Then such things as the child's age, body size, the size and shape of his external ears, and the dimensions of the ear canal must be taken into account. Among factors to be considered are the conditions under which the hearing aids will be worn; the relative cost and reliability of suitable instruments; the cost of running the hearing aid (batteries, parts); and the availability, cost, speed, and quality of service. At some time, all hearing aids need repair. The experience of the audiologists, teacher/clinicians, and other parents with local hearing aid dealers can be of help in some of these respects. They may be able to direct a "new" parent to one of the many dealers who go out of their way to help children and take a personal interest in their progress.

Amplification

Hearing aids all provide some degree of gain (amplification) over a range of frequencies. They differ in the amount of gain they provide, in the range of frequencies over which they amplify, in the relative amount of amplification they provide for low- and high-frequency sounds, and in the maximum amount of power they can deliver. Some incorporate controls that permit the adjustment of all of the characteristics mentioned above. Others have few, if any, such controls.

Gain is the amount by which a hearing aid increases the intensity of a sound. Gain may be measured at 1000 Hz, the approximate center frequency of speech, at the three frequencies 1000, 1600, and 2500 Hz (average high frequency [HF] gain), or at the point in the frequency range where it provides most amplification (peak gain). All these measures have value, but no one measure offers more than a guideline in selecting an appropriate instrument for a given child. Hearing-impaired children need gain in the frequency range where it helps them most. This may not be at any of the points mentioned above.

The *frequency range* of a hearing aid is normally calculated through reference to a chart showing the instrument's frequency response, that is, its gain at various frequencies. Such a chart is shown as Figure 6.2. To make such a chart, one must place the hearing aid in a small sound-proof box into which a test tone of a certain intensity (the input) is introduced. The receiver of the hearing aid is coupled to a device that records the sound level produced (the output) when the test tone is changed in frequency from under 100 Hz to over 8000 Hz. Using such a chart, the gain (output minus input) can be calculated for any or all frequencies tested. Usually, the frequency range of a hearing aid is considered to lie between the two points where a horizontal line—drawn 20 dB below the average of its gain provided at 1000, 1600 and 2500 Hz—intersects the curve drawn on the chart. The frequency range of the hearing aid used to produce Figure 6.2 was 375 to 3000 Hz. Calculating the frequency range in this way can be misleading because many children with residual hearing in the low frequencies can hear sounds reproduced by the hearing aid below that range. Similarly, some children may be able to hear sounds that the hearing aid amplifies above that range.

The saturation sound pressure level (SSPL 90) of a hearing aid must also be determined. Beyond this level, formerly described as maximum power output (MPO), no increase in output intensity will be caused by increasing input levels. Normally, input + gain = output. Thus, with a 60 dB input and a gain of 40 dB, the output will be 100 dB; with an input of 60 dB and a gain of 60 dB, the output will be 120 dB. Suppose, however, that the SSPL of a hearing aid is limited to 100 dB. In this case, with an input level of 60 dB, the hearing aid could provide no more than 40 dB gain before reaching saturation output level. The SSPL of a hearing aid is as important as its gain, for just as the hearing aid would be of no use to the child if it had insufficient gain to raise speech to an audible level, so would its value be limited if it made certain sounds too loud for the child to tolerate.

Distortion may be present in a hearing aid. It is important to check for distortion because an instrument that deforms sounds in the process of amplifying them may make it harder for the child to learn to use his hearing. Several forms of distortion may be present in a hearing aid. Those most commonly encountered are harmonic distortion, intermodulation distortion, transient distortion, and circuit noise. Harmonic distortion occurs when one tone at a given frequency, say 500 Hz, is presented at the microphone and several tones such as 500, 1000, and 1500 Hz are reproduced at the receiver. Intermodulation distortion occurs when two tones presented at the microphone interact and thus cause other tones to be reproduced at the receiver. Transient distortion occurs when the durational aspects of a sound are radically changed through the process of amplification. A hearing aid which causes transient distortion may make the word "sip" sound like "tip," or the word "chip" sound like "dip." Any of these forms of distortion can be due to a fault in the microphone, the amplifier, or the receiver. Such problems often arise either when the hearing aid's batteries have little power left in them, or when the aid has been dropped and one or other of its components damaged. Distortion is not usually severe enough to be of concern in new instruments, but since it can arise through the hard wear and tear to which children subject hearing aids, listening for distortion and undue circuit noise should be part of the daily checking procedure. We shall discuss such procedures later in this chapter.

Figure 6.2 (opposite):
The response of a hearing aid typical of those used by severely hearing-impaired children. Gain at each frequency can be calculated by subtracting 70 dB (the input level) from the output level depicted by the curve.

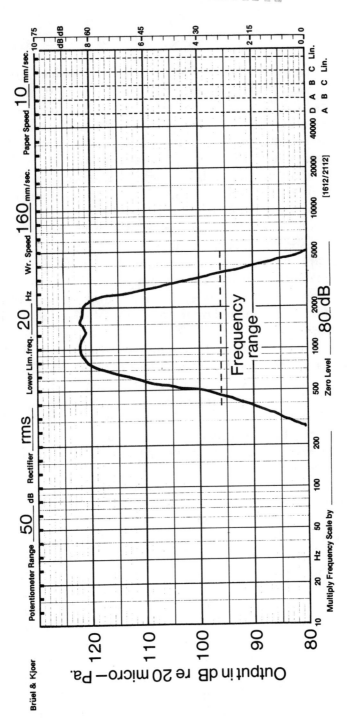

Hearing Aid Selection

The selection of a hearing aid is not a precise scientific procedure. It typically involves the use of approximate data, educated guesswork, and finally compromise. Even when the most appropriate hearing aids have been selected for a given child, they are unlikely to compensate fully for his hearing impairment. Eyeglasses can usually help children with faulty vision to see much more effectively than hearing aids can help hearing-impaired children to hear. In spite of these facts, hearing aid selection is not an entirely hit-or-miss affair, and hearing aids remain the most effective tool a child can use in acquiring spoken language skills.

The first step in selecting a hearing aid for a child is to determine the approximate gain and frequency range required. These can be calculated by using information derived from two sources: the audiologic assessment (see Chapter 5) and the body of knowledge that has accumulated on the acoustics of speech (see Chapter 4). Children who are considered to be candidates for hearing aid use are already known to be hearing-impaired, and their thresholds of detection have been closely estimated. The approximate intensity and frequency range of speech sounds can also be specified. The least amount of gain required can therefore be derived by calculating how much amplification is needed to raise the intensity of the various speech sounds to levels that would render them audible to the child. The optimal amount of gain required cannot be determined so readily.

If sounds are to be discriminable—more than just audible— they must reach the ear at levels above threshold. One can only guess how much above threshold levels speech has to be in order that words can be discriminated, identified, and understood. It follows that threshold measures can be no more than a guide, and therefore it does not make sense to wait until a reliable audiogram is obtained before one provides a young child with a hearing aid. Valuable listening time would be needlessly lost if one waited until test after test proved that initial audiograms were reliable to within a few decibels. In most cases, it would be unrealistic to attempt to ascertain required gain to within such fine limits. The average level of the speech signal commonly varies with distance and from speaker to speaker by at least 20 dB. Relatively gross estimates of threshold will therefore usually serve in initial selection procedures.

The second step in hearing aid selection is to determine the child's approximate loudness discomfort level (LDL)—the level at which sounds are too powerful to be easily tolerated. Listening to speech should be a pleasant experience. Hearing aids should therefore raise the intensity levels of speech sounds so that they are audible, but not raise them to the extent that they—or other sounds—become annoyingly loud. There is no single, generally accepted, measure for determining loudness discomfort levels in children. They can, however, be subjectively judged by careful observation of a child's responses to noises of different types. Noises with sharp onset like a handclap, one castanet struck against another, or a syllable such as [ba] spoken in a loud voice close to the microphone are quite effective stimuli for such a test. They have characteristics in common with the environmental sounds that most disturb hearing aid users.

The difference between the threshold of detection for sound and the loudness discomfort level is known as the dynamic range of hearing. If a child's loudness discomfort level is about 110 dB and his average threshold is 50 dB, his dynamic range would be 60 dB (110–50). Since the dynamic range of speech—from the loudest vowel to the quietest consonant—is about 30 dB, a child with a 60 dB dynamic range of hearing should have no problem in receiving all speech sounds comfortably with one of many available hearing aids. The more restricted the child's dynamic range of hearing, the more difficult it is to find a hearing aid that suits his needs. Hearing aids are available that amplify the louder sounds less than the quieter sounds and thus compress the dynamic range of speech. Aids that function in this fashion incorporate a feature known as automatic volume control (AVC), or automatic gain control (AGC). Research to improve the way in which hearing aids compress sound is in progress. One aspect of this research is concerned with the possibilities offered by building several compression circuits into one hearing aid so that sounds in certain frequency bands are compressed or amplified more than others.

In the preceding discussion we have related intensity of sound to audiometric zero, the threshold of detection of normal listeners. Intensity in decibels above audiometric zero is specified as dB HL (hearing level). Engineers who produce and measure hearing aids relate the output of hearing aids to different reference points, namely, 0.0002 dynes per square centimeter or 20 micropascals. Intensity in decibels above this reference point is specified as dB SPL. (These initials stand for sound pressure level.) The human ear is not so sensitive to sounds at low and high frequencies as it is to sounds in the mid-frequency range; yet even in mid-frequency range, sound at 0 dB SPL usually cannot be heard. The difference between dB SPL and dB HL at the various frequencies on the audiogram was specified in 1969 by the American National Standards Institute (ANSI) as follows: 125 Hz, 43 dB; 250 Hz, 25 dB; 500 Hz, 11.5 dB; 1000 Hz, 7 dB; 2000 Hz, 9 dB; 4000 Hz, 9.5 dB, and 8000 Hz, 13 dB. This means that the normal human ear is less sensitive than the engineers' reference point at each of these frequencies by the number of decibels indicated above. Because this is so, hearing aids with a maximum power output of 130 dB SPL over the center frequencies would, in fact, reproduce sound no louder than 118.5 dB HL at 500 Hz, 123 dB HL at 1000 Hz, and 121 dB HL at 2000 Hz.

The fact that dB SPL and dB HL are both used in audiology often causes confusion. Confusion can be avoided, however, if the reader remembers that whether one calculates gain in dB SPL or dB HL, the result is the same. Most texts on hearing aid selection attempt to clarify the task by calculating required gain as engineers do, using charts showing dB SPL. We shall do the reverse, and illustrate selection procedures by referring to dB HL and using the audiogram as our guide through the following steps:

First, we depict a representative range of speech sounds on the audiogram form (see Figure 6.3). The sounds we use are the vowels [u], [a], [i] and the consonants [ʃ] and [s] as normally spoken by an adult male at a distance of two yards. These sounds include low-, mid-, and high-frequency components of speech, and ability to hear all five of these sounds implies ability to hear all other sounds of speech.

Second, we chart the child's threshold on the same form. Typical responses of a child with moderate hearing impairment are also shown in Figure 6.3.

Third, we calculate the difference between the speech sounds and the thresholds obtained at each of the five frequencies 250 through 4000 Hz. These differences represent the *least* gain required to render speech audible.

Fourth, we chart the child's loudness discomfort level (LDL) or, if responses indicating discomfort cannot be obtained, we assume a discomfort level of 120 dB (see Figure 6.3).

Fifth, we add half the value of the child's dynamic range of hearing at each of the five frequencies 250 through 4000 Hz to the least gain requirements calculated in our third step. The figures obtained represent approximate optimal gain at each of these frequencies. In the case of the child whose data are provided in Figure 6.3, these figures are 250 Hz, 50 dB; 500 Hz, 50 dB;

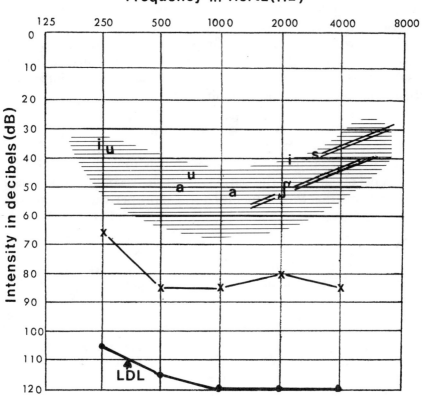

Figure 6.3

An audiogram form showing the relative intensity levels (HL) of the main components of the five sounds [u, a, i, ʃ, s] spoken at two yards. By calculating how much amplification is required to increase these sounds so that they fall between the child's threshold of hearing and his loudness discomfort level (LDL), one can calculate the approximate gain that should be provided by a hearing aid.

1000 Hz, 55 dB; 2000 Hz, 55 dB, and 4000 Hz, 70 dB gain.*

Sixth, we repeat the procedure to calculate amplification requirements for the child's other ear. With children who have some spoken language skills we check the validity of our calculations by carrying out speech tests of hearing on a master hearing aid, an instrument that allows one to simulate the characteristics of a variety of individual hearing aids.

Seventh, we identify the body-worn or head-worn hearing aids that will provide the gain and frequency response desired. Since we recognize that the procedures we have used (like the procedures any other workers would use) can yield only approximate specification of need, we look for instruments that permit some adjustment of maximum gain, maximum output, frequency response, and compression.

Eighth, we recommend that the parents obtain the appropriate earmolds and arrange to have specific instruments on trial from a dealer. If the parents agree, we contact the dealer to introduce them and to describe their requirements.

Hearing Aid Fitting

The initial step in fitting hearing aids is to verify that the instruments obtained by the parents meet the recommended specifications, and that the earmolds conform properly to the contours

---

*Note that a hearing aid with gain characteristics as selected by this procedure would be close to the child's amplification requirements for listening in quiet conditions. However, noise pervades one's life. To counteract the effect of noise, which is predominantly found in the low-frequency range, amplification below 1000 Hz has to be reduced as far as possible, i.e., to the point where further reduction would render low-frequency cues inaudible. One has no problem in this respect for the child whose audiogram is shown in Figure 6.3. He has a sufficiently large dynamic range for gain in the frequencies above 1000 Hz to be increased, and for gain in the lower frequencies to be reduced. The amount of gain provided at or below 250 Hz is not such an important factor in masking as the difference in gain for frequencies below 250 Hz and above 1000 Hz. Under most conditions, a difference of about 20 dB will prevent upward spread of masking and yet conserve audibility of low-frequency acoustic cues.

of the ears. The check on the hearing aids is carried out using test equipment that measures frequency response. The check on the earmolds calls first for visual inspection and second for confirmation that there is no acoustic howl (feedback) when the hearing aids are worn at the required gain setting.

Placing the hearing aids on the child and adjusting them is a procedure that requires previous planning. Hearing aids will initially feel strange to the child, and the natural tendency of any child is to reject the strange and unfamiliar. Rejection is particularly likely to occur if the adults involved appear to be dubious about the outcome of the procedure. The parent and the teacher/clinician concerned should therefore approach the initial fitting calmly and with confidence. They should show pleasure in putting the hearing aids on the child and indicate that they expect him to enjoy the experience. Prior counseling should help parents feel and act positively and genuinely in this situation. Even given a positive attitude on the part of the adults, the strangeness of wearing earmolds is likely to lead to the child pulling them out unless his attention is drawn to something of stronger interest. New toys and activities should therefore be available to distract the child as soon as the initial fitting is accomplished.

Some workers recommend that hearing aids should be worn for a few minutes the first day, longer periods the next, and longer periods still on subsequent days so that the child gradually comes to accept the instruments. In our experience, this procedure often leads to long delays in establishing full-time usage. Rather as one's tongue wanders to the cavity caused by a lost filling in a tooth and renewed attention to the tooth when the cavity is filled, so will a child be made overconscious and unaccepting of the hearing aids if they are frequently put on and taken off. We have found it better to expect acceptance and full-time usage within the first week (or ten days).

As soon as the child is sufficiently used to his hearing aids, the validity of the selection must be checked. The procedure described in selecting the instruments was theoretical and based on threshold measures. The child's actual ability to detect and discriminate speech with the aids selected—as they were delivered and as they can be adjusted—must therefore be determined as soon as possible after the child's initial acceptance of the instruments and their regular use.

Detection of Amplified Speech

To determine whether the child can detect the expected range of speech sounds, we also employ as stimuli the five sounds [u, a, i, ʃ and s]. The acoustic patterns of these sounds are depicted in Figure 6.3. With a baby, one can determine whether the sounds are audible by means of behavioral testing, in which the child is reinforced for responding (as described in Chapter 5). The older child can be asked to raise a finger or clap his hands when the sound is heard. Children with measurable hearing up to 1000 Hz and appropriate amplification should be able to hear the three vowels spoken in a quiet voice at a distance of at least five yards. Children with hearing up to 2000 Hz should hear the [ʃ] equally well. Those with hearing up to 4000 Hz should be able to detect the [s] from at least two yards if their thresholds for this frequency do not exceed 80 dB. With older children, one can carry out the test in low-frequency noise to determine whether there is too much amplification of the low frequencies. If such is the case, upward spread of masking will occur, and the consonants will be less audible in noise than in quiet.

The suprasegmental aspects of speech—rhythm, intonation, stress—are principally carried by the vowels and voiced sounds in speech. If the three vowels in the five-sound test, described above, can be heard, one can therefore be certain that suprasegmental patterns will also be audible to the child. If the [ʃ] can be heard, then the second formant (F_2) of [i] will also be audible since it falls in the same frequency range at a comparable intensity (see Figure 6.3). Hearing for [ʃ] implies that the child will be able to discriminate [u] and [i], which have similar first formants (F_1). If the [u] is audible and the [i] is not, then poor high-frequency hearing and inadequate gain for the low frequencies are indicated. Since [u] and [i] have first formants in the same frequency range, ability to hear [u] but not [i] is evidence that the child is responding to the second formant of [u]. If the child can hear only the [a] vowel, gain below 1000 Hz is inadequate, since both F_1 and F_2 of [u] and F_1 of [i] lie below this frequency. Inability to hear the [s] indicates either insufficient gain in the high frequencies or absence of hearing around 4000 Hz. These points may be deduced from the information provided in Chapter 4 and above.

Parents and professionals should regularly check the hearing aids children use by listening to the way they amplify the five sounds [u, a, i, ʃ, s]. When these sounds are not adequately amplified or when their reproduction is distorted, the hearing aid should be serviced. If a normal-hearing listener cannot hear a sound through a hearing aid, then the child cannot be expected to detect it either. One must be as concerned with the quality of amplification the child is receiving as with the amount of gain provided. Checking whether the aid works simply by turning it on to see if it produces feedback is not adequate.

Discrimination of Amplified Speech

Evidence that the child can discriminate between or among particular speech sounds is provided only when he responds differentially to unlike stimuli. Any reliable response is acceptable as evidence that a sound is audible, but in tests of discrimination the child must either say the sounds compared, press one button rather than another, or point to one particular picture or object in a given set. The child's age and abilities will largely determine how his speech discrimination skills can be judged.

Speech discrimination is not an all-or-none affair. Speech patterns can differ from each other in many ways (see Chapter 4). Some suprasegmental contrasts—such as high/low, loud/quiet, long/short, and many vs. few syllables —are of considerable magnitude and demand only gross discrimination skill. Segmental contrasts—differences between phonemes—vary in magnitude according to the number of manner, place, and voicing features that render them distinct. Thus the consonants in the syllables [ma] and [sa] differ in manner, place, and voicing. They are highly contrastive, whereas the consonants in the syllables [fa] and [sa] are less so, differing only in place of production. Of course, speech patterns in which both the suprasegmental and segmental patterns differ offer most contrast. It is therefore essential in testing discrimination of segmental patterns to hold suprasegmental patterns constant, and vice-versa.

Speech patterns must be clearly audible if they are to be discriminated one from another. Such a statement might appear trite, yet failure to recognize this may trap the unwary. For example, a child may respond differentially to the [ʃa] and [sa], and do so not because he hears both consonants but because the [ʃ] is audible and the [s] inaudible. Similarly, two sounds may be audible, but one or both may have components that lie below or too close to threshold to permit discrimination. Such might be the case with the vowels [u] and [i] if the second formant of [i], which lies between 2000 and 3000 Hz, is amplified insufficiently for the child with hearing in this band of frequencies. A further example is provided by considering the common confusion of [m] and [b] by hearing-impaired children. Both sounds may be audible to a child, but if the hearing aid provides little or no gain in the 200–300 Hz range, the low-frequency murmur and first formant consonant-to-vowel transitions characteristic of nasal consonants will not be available to him. Auditory confusion of the [m] and [b] in a variety of vowel contexts might be expected if such is the case.

Adjustment of the frequency response of hearing aids with a view to improving the child's speech discrimination capacity is part of hearing aid fitting. By such means, many auditory confusions such as those mentioned above can be prevented. Adjustment may be carried out as part of a clinical evaluation session by an audiologist working with children who have sufficient spoken language skills to respond to a standardized speech discrimination test and/or to a series of paired sound discriminations. Standardized speech discrimination tests can be used to obtain scores (items correct) which allow the comparison of one child or group of children with another. For the purpose of hearing aid fitting, however, the analysis of errors (confusions) made on such a test is as important as the number of items correct. Error analysis allows one to identify the types of sound with which the child has difficulty, to determine whether there is consistent confusion of one sound or class of sounds with another, and to discover whether changing the frequency response of the hearing aid leads to a reduction in particular types of confusion. A paired sound discrimination task can be used either as a supplement or as an alternative to such testing. In this type of task, the child's ability to differentiate syllables that contain contrasting features is determined. Thus one pair, such as [ba-ma], is used to test nasal/plosive discrimination. Another pair, such as [da-ga], is used to test place discrimination, and so on. Dozens of different pairs are, of course, required to identify those sounds which are consistently discriminated from others and those which are confused.

Adjustment of hearing aids on the basis of speech discrimination ability can rarely be made through the clinical testing of very young children who have little or no spoken language skill. Data on the child's ability to discriminate can usually be gleaned only in the course of observations and tests carried out as his training proceeds and as he learns what discriminations are important and how to make them. Effective early training, competent data gathering, and adequate hearing aid fitting for the pre-verbal child demand that the teacher/clinicians employed with young children be thoroughly familiar with training and testing procedures, with the acoustics of speech, and with hearing aids.

Speech sound discrimination has been tested in many normally hearing infants under 6 months of age. Changes in the rate at which the infant sucks, or changes in his heart rate, for example, can often be recorded when a different consonant is introduced in a series of syllables. Imagine the baby quietly listening to [bababa-ba . . .] and his reaction when the syllable is changed to [dadada-da . . .]. Just as one habituates to a clock ticking and becomes suddenly aware of the silence when it stops, so does the baby who can discriminate between a pair of sounds become aware that a different consonant has been substituted. Paired sound discrimination tasks of this type might well be used clinically with hearing-impaired children. Such work and its applicability in the fitting of hearing aids remains for future workers to investigate.

Earmolds

The purpose of an earmold is to direct the output of the hearing aid into the ear canal. Thus all earmolds have a channel (a hole bored through them) leading from the receiver into the ear canal. Earmolds can significantly change the acoustic pattern delivered by the hearing aid. For example, as much as 15–20 dB of the gain a hearing aid provides for the low frequencies can be lost if the earmold does not fit snugly enough to form a good acoustic seal; and peaks or troughs in the frequency response curve of the hearing aid can be shifted in frequency according to how much of the ear canal is occupied by the earmold. The case for adjusting the hearing aid as part of the fitting procedure rests partly on facts such as these.

Full or complete earmolds—those that completely block the ear canal except for the channel leading to the receiver—also act as earplugs. Only the sounds reproduced by the aid can enter the ear canals unhindered by such earmolds. Other sounds are either excluded or attenuated. Such a situation is not always desirable. Some children with moderate high-frequency hearing loss might benefit from listening to both unamplified low-frequency sounds and amplified high-frequency sounds. Vented or open earmolds can be provided for such cases. Vented molds are so called because a further channel leading from the ear canal directly to the outer surface of the earmold is bored through the material. Open earmolds simply hold the tubing from the hearing aid receiver in position, and leave most of the entrance to the ear canal open. Vented and open earmolds allow both amplified and unamplified sound to enter the ear canal. Ear-level hearing aids with output levels greater than about 100 dB cannot be coupled to the ear with such earmolds because sound leaking back from the ear canal into the microphone of the hearing aid will cause acoustic feedback—a whistle or a howl.

Acoustic feedback can also occur with full earmolds that do not fit snugly into the ear canal. The fit of the earmold is crucially important if head-level hearing aids providing output levels of more than 115 dB are to be considered. Children's ears grow, and earmolds can eventually fit slackly as a result. It may therefore be very difficult, if not impossible, for certain children—mainly those who need high levels of amplification—to wear head-level hearing aids without acoustic feedback. Hearing aids amplify speech in a distorted form, if at all, when such feedback occurs. The alternatives for children who have acoustic feedback problems with head-level hearing aids are new earmolds, or body-worn hearing aids. Reducing gain to the point where acoustic feedback disappears is no solution to the problem. Under such a condition the child's amplification needs will simply not be met.

New earmolds may provide but a temporary solution to an acoustic feedback problem. Once the ears grow again, the problem will recur. If new, close-fitting earmolds can be successfully obtained as soon and as often as feedback is noticed, then there is no need to consider body-worn instruments. Head-level hearing aids can produce as much gain and as wide a frequency range as body-worn instruments. They are preferable to body-worn instruments on several counts: head-level aids are cosmetically more appealing; they provide better potential for localization of sound; they produce sound free from clothes rub (a problem that causes considerable masking in body-worn instruments); and their position renders them less likely to be damaged by water or other fluids that tend to fall onto the microphone or controls of body-worn instruments. These potential advantages cannot be realized if feedback consistently occurs. Technology has not yet advanced to the stage where feedback can be eliminated by improved circuitry (although such improvements are feasible). The more widespread use of head-level hearing aids at the present time therefore depends mainly on the provision of more satisfactory earmolds.

Body-worn hearing aids are not so prone to feedback as head-level instruments because the microphone is usually located further—indeed, several inches—from the ear. Earmolds that provide a relatively poor seal may, therefore, cause no acoustic feedback when used with body-worn hearing aids. Acoustic feedback does, of course, occur with high-power body-worn instruments, but usually the earmold is at fault.

Earmolds may be hard or soft. Tightly fitting hard earmolds, if they project well into the ear canal, may cause the child discomfort or work loose when he eats or talks. The jawbone (mandible) tends to move and dislodge hard earmolds during such activities. Soft earmolds are more likely to bend as the jaw moves and stay firmly in place. Soft earmolds are also less likely to cut or bruise a child should the child suffer a blow to the ear in sports or through a fall. We once counted the number of days during a school year that two groups of 10 children were unable to wear hearing aids due to ear damage. We found that, due to cuts and bruises, all of those who had hard earmolds were unable to use hearing aids for periods ranging from one to five weeks. A few with soft earmolds missed one or two days on this account, but most, none at all.

Binaural Versus Monaural Amplification

Binaural listening is superior to monaural listening for several reasons. The ability to hear with two ears rather than one allows listeners to localize the source of speech and hence to turn to face the speaker; to hear equally well whether speech arrives from one side of the head or the other; and to hear better in the presence of background noise and to listen with less effort. These advantages, enjoyed by normal-hearing listeners, have also been demonstrated for subjects who wear binaural hearing aids. They cannot be demonstrated when one hearing aid is used to drive two receivers. Throughout this chapter we have consistently treated hearing aid selection and fitting for two ears rather than one. In part, our preference for binaural hearing aids stems from recognition of the advantages specified above. There are, however, at least three additional reasons for recommending binaural amplification for most hearing-impaired listeners.

First, audiograms show that most hearing-impaired children have similar, but not identical, thresholds in their two ears. Thus, at one frequency, the threshold in the right ear may be better than that in the left by 5 to 10 dB. At other frequencies the reverse might be true. Now, if two hearing aids are used, the child's threshold responses at each frequency will be those of the ear that has the better thresholds: The two ears, in short, can complement each other.

Second, a sound presented at a given intensity to two ears is heard as louder than the same sound presented to one ear. This "binaural summation" effect allows one to listen comfortably with two ears at lower intensity levels than with one ear. Children therefore require less output from two hearing aids than from one aid to reach a comfortable listening level. Since increase in hearing impairment can be caused by wearing over-powerful hearing aids, the reduction of power requirements obtained through binaural as compared with monaural amplification lessens the risk of additional hearing loss. Although this risk is negligible with hearing aids having moderate (30–40 dB) gain and output levels of less than 120 dB, it increases with the use of more powerful instruments. Hearing aids with maximum output levels exceeding 130 dB are quite likely to cause further deterioration of hearing.

Third, the two hemispheres of the brain have specialized functions. The right hemisphere, principally served by the left ear, normally processes nonverbal, spatial material; whereas the left hemisphere, principally served by the right ear, usually processes verbal material. Material received by the ears is integrated, and signals from either ear can reach both hemispheres. Less information reaches the brain, however, if only one ear is operational. Optimal development of the brain's specialized capacities is therefore more likely to be fostered by the use of two ears rather than one. Even when hearing impairment in the two ears is substantially different, there is more opportunity for the brain to develop its specialized capacities and to integrate the signals received from each ear. If only the high-frequency sounds in a message are presented to one ear and only the low-frequency sounds of that message are presented to the other, the brain is capable of fusing the two different but related signals into a meaningful whole.

There are strong parallels between binaural versus monaural hearing and binocular versus monocular vision. Consider reading. It is normally possible to read equally as well (but perhaps not so easily) with one eye or the other as with two. The task does not demand the very thing that binocular vision can provide, namely depth perception. Try to thread a needle using one eye as compared with two. Because depth perception is involved, the task is much easier when both eyes are employed. There are also many listening tasks that can be carried out as effectively with one ear as with two. Several studies of binaural hearing aids have employed such tasks and hence have not demonstrated the advantages that accrue to using two ears. Given that these advantages can be demonstrated, should binaural hearing aids be worn by all hearing-impaired children?

To suggest that all hearing-impaired children should wear binaural hearing aids would be irrational. Without question, the hearing aid selection and fitting procedures outlined in this chapter would identify certain (relatively rare) children who could hear better monaurally than binaurally. Clearly such children should wear one aid rather than two. Similarly, the procedures mentioned above would also demonstrate that certain children could not benefit from hearing aids at all. They should not be expected to wear them. An auditory-oral approach cannot be used with such children. Let us stress, however, that our procedures are pragmatic. We do not have blind faith in clinical assessments, but require that the results of such assessments be extended and confirmed in the course of ongoing diagnostic training of the individual child. Only with the evidence obtained in the course of such training—training that requires hearing aid use during all waking hours—would we accept that one hearing aid is better for a given child than two.

Maintenance and Routine Checks

The maintenance of a child's hearing aids is a task that requires at least daily attention from the parents with periodic checks by the teacher/clinician or audiologist. Parents should ensure that batteries have sufficient power, that the cords of body-worn hearing aids are in good condition, that the receivers have suffered no evident damage, and that the hearing aid reproduces speech as it is supposed to. The different checks that are required are briefly described below.

Batteries are best checked in the evening, after a full day's use, preferably with a volt meter. If checked in the morning, batteries may have temporarily recovered their voltage and the capacity of the battery to last a whole day may be misjudged. Batteries should be the first thing checked if a hearing aid does not work. Batteries that are almost exhausted may supply sufficient power for the hearing aid to operate, but not to amplify without distortion. They should therefore be discarded as soon as their voltage drops below the level prescribed in the handbook supplied with each hearing aid. The length of time batteries will last depends on the type of cell used, the power requirements of the hearing aid, and how long the aid is used each day. Manufacturers specify the type of cells that can be used with a given hearing aid and their expected life in hours. The life expectancy and cost of batteries required should certainly be considered when hearing aids are selected.

Cords of body-worn hearing aids break quite readily because they are exposed to considerable wear and tear during a child's normal daily activities. If the batteries are in good order and the aid does not work, the cord should be replaced as a first step in fault location. Cords may be fractured rather than broken. As part of the daily check, the receiver can be placed against the microphone and the cord shaken. Fractured cords will cause the feedback to become intermittent—rather like a Morse code signal. Speech through hearing aids with such a problem will also be intermittent, so the cord should be replaced. Various lengths of cord are available, and a supply of spare cords selected to suit the size of the child should always be kept in stock by the parents and the teacher/clinician working with the child.

Receivers of body-worn hearing aids are also prone to frequent damage and should be checked daily. The casing should be examined for cracks, and the washer interposed between the earmold and the receiver should be tested for snugness of fit. If the earmold is loosely coupled to the receiver, feedback may readily occur. If cords and batteries are known to be in good condition and the hearing aid does not work, a new receiver should be tried. If the aid does not then function, internal damage may be assumed. External receivers similar to those used with body-worn hearing aids may be used with head-level instruments. A variety of receivers may be used with a particular hearing aid. Usually, the frequency response of the hearing aid can be radically changed by using different receivers. A particular receiver is usually chosen for the child as part of the hearing aid selection and fitting procedure described above. A few spare receivers of the chosen type should therefore be kept on hand so that broken or damaged receivers can be replaced.

Internal damage to the hearing aid or to an external receiver may not result in complete breakdown but may, instead, cause distortion of one sort or another. A complete daily check must therefore include listening for such distortion. It is not enough to verify that feedback occurs when the instrument is switched on. We have found that listening to the five sounds [u, a, i, ʃ and s] through the hearing aid can quickly indicate the presence of significant distortion. An earmold should be used by the person making this check. The test is best made at the gain settings normally used by the child. The three vowels should be reproduced at similar levels of intensity, and the sounds [ʃ] and [s] should be clearly heard. By listening consistently to these five sounds from the time the hearing aid is obtained, one becomes so familiar with their patterns that any radical change in frequency response will be easily detected. Gradual change in the quality of the sound reproduced by a hearing aid is much more difficult to notice. This is one reason why periodic, objective testing of any instrument is strongly recommended. One indication that a change in the frequency response of a hearing aid has gradually occurred is that the child uses a different gain control setting.

Once an effective gain control setting on a well-fitted hearing aid has been determined, any major adjustment made by the child indicates that something in his auditory system has changed. It might be the hearing aid, the presence of an ear infection, or the child's ability to process sound more effectively as the result of training. Whatever the reason, such adjustments indicate that an objective hearing aid evaluation, a thorough audiologic assessment, or both are required.

Evaluation and assessments should not be scheduled rigidly on a yearly basis. Problems and faults are not annual events. They can develop at any time during the child's training. Evaluation and assessments should therefore be scheduled on demand, as the teacher/clinician or parent requests them to meet a child's immediate need. Such requests will not be made lightly by a competent person.

A common problem that we have discovered in hearing aids that have been dropped or otherwise damaged is that they develop a peak in frequency response at or near 1000 Hz. A peak in this frequency range is particularly noxious because the greatest amount of masking occurs in the frequency range just above the masking sound. Since the crucial information on place of consonant production is carried in the frequency range 1500–3200 Hz, peaks of gain just below this region serve to emphasize the relatively strong second formants of central vowels and mask such information. It is surprising that some manufacturers produce new hearing aids with peaks in response at or near 1000 Hz. One can only assume that their engineers know little about hearing and speech acoustics.

Peaks of gain at or around 1000 Hz may also cause a child to reduce the gain of his hearing aid (see above) in order to prevent

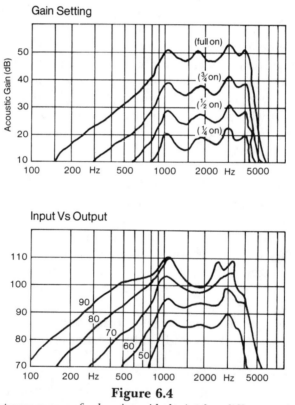

Figure 6.4

Frequency response curves of a hearing aid obtained at different gain and input settings. The figure shows the loss of frequency range (horizontal axis) that occurs as gain (vertical axis) is reduced.

sounds from reaching his loudness discomfort level. In doing so, he may reduce the amplification actually required for the detection and discrimination of sounds higher or lower in frequency. Reducing the gain of a hearing aid also reduces its effective frequency range. This effect is clearly demonstrated in Figure 6.4. Note that when gain (vertical axis) is reduced by about 10 dB, the frequency range (horizontal axis) is reduced by at least 200 Hz. A reduction of 10 dB can thus reduce frequency range so that low formants of [u] and [i] and the typical low-frequency murmur of nasal consonants become inaudible to the child for whom such an aid at full gain is adequate.

Tolerance problems, perhaps caused by peaks in the response of the hearing aid, often lead to older hearing-impaired children turning off their hearing aids or keeping gain to a minimum and inadequate level. Turning the hearing aid down or off may equally well indicate that the child regards the use of residual hearing as unimportant. It occurs most often among children who receive too little meaningful auditory stimulation and who are not consistently expected to listen, or who did not receive hearing aids in early childhood. In such cases the remedy lies with the parents and the teacher/clinician rather than with the audiologist and the hearing aid.

ANNOTATED BIBLIOGRAPHY

Berger, K. W.   *The Hearing Aid: Its Operation and Development.* Michigan: National Hearing Aid Society, 1970.
A book that traces the technological developments that have led to modern, miniaturized hearing aids, this volume is for those who are primarily interested in instrumentation.

Ling, D.   Conventional hearing aids: an overview. *The Volta Review*, (73, 343–352, 375–383, 1971).
It provides a brief analysis of amplification needs of hearing-impaired children and how they can best be met. Available in reprint form, it is an inexpensive introductory paper that provides more than one hundred references to books and articles and, in spite of its publication date, can be considered as current material.

Miller, M.   *Hearing Aids.* Indianapolis: The Bobbs Merrill Co., 1972.

This is a small, inexpensive booklet in the Bobbs Merrill Series in communicative disorders. It is easy to read and provides an excellent introduction to the topic of amplification.

Pollack, M. C. (Ed.)   *Amplification for the Hearing-Impaired.* New York: Grune and Stratton, 1975.

No publication on hearing aids is more comprehensive than this one. It includes chapters on various aspects of amplification by many leading experts, all of whom write clearly and with the utmost authority on their topics. All provide key references to other material. The majority of texts on audiology contain chapters on hearing aids, but this one brings knowledge in the field into perspective in one text.

7. The Use of Residual Hearing

*O*ptimal use of residual hearing is difficult to achieve. Few hearing aids provide entirely satisfactory amplification, and the acoustic conditions in which they have to be used are rarely ideal. Because the child does not always react overtly to sounds that he can hear—and one cannot expect him to do so—direct and immediate measures of speech reception are not always available. Speech reception depends heavily upon a child's linguistic skills, yet the body of scientific knowledge on language comprehension is relatively small. In spite of such problems, certain principles underlying the use of residual hearing have emerged. This chapter will be concerned mainly with such principles, knowledge of which is essential if high levels of speech and language are to be achieved.

Historical Perspective

For several hundred years, isolated reports of teachers who have used their children's residual hearing have appeared in the literature relating to hearing impairment. It was not until the end of the last century, however, that the use of residual hearing became relatively common in the education of hearing-impaired children. Ear trumpets, which concentrated and conducted sound into the ear canal, were then in relatively common use among adults; and speaking tubes, which conducted the teacher's speech directly to the child's ear, were frequently used in schools for the deaf. Speaking tubes connected together were also used to teach small classes of children. The use of such equipment persisted

111

until about 50 years ago, when electronic hearing aids became generally available.

The first electronic hearing aids were large, heavy instruments. Not being portable, they were used exclusively in classrooms or clinics. The teacher/clinician spoke into a free-standing microphone and the hearing-impaired listener(s) received the amplified sound through headphones. These early electronic aids revolutionized life opportunities for many children. Since such aids provided more powerful amplification than speaking tubes, children who were more severely hearing impaired could benefit from them.

The history of hearing aids is fascinating. Their development has reflected the advances made in other areas of technology — advances which have lifted man from the earth to the moon. Knowledge of the origin of these advances helps us to understand why certain present-day notions and practices relative to hearing aids and their use exist. Time-honored practices were not wholly unsatisfactory, and inertia inevitably prevents speedy and widespread adoption of new technology, its products and applications. Consider the following examples: (1) Binaural fittings were impossible with the cumbersome instruments available in the 1940s. Monaural fitting therefore became an established practice, and even now inertia (plus cost) has made it difficult for many people to accept the fact that binaural fitting is truly preferable. (2) Body-worn hearing aids appeared before miniaturization allowed head-level instruments to be developed. Nevertheless, many children who could wear head-level instruments are currently fitted with body-worn hearing aids (some, of course, need them). (3) Because lessons in auditory discrimination were devised for the formal training of children on group hearing aids, many people still consider "auditory training" a self-contained subject to be taught. It was not uncommon, until recently, for the training of children in schools for the deaf to be limited to lessons on a group hearing aid for an hour or two each week.

Only during the past few decades have hearing aids become small enough for children to wear them continuously—all day and every day. Wearable hearing aids provided the opportunity for hearing-impaired children to have something better and more extensive than auditory training—namely, auditory experience in real-life situations. It is in such situations that spoken language skills are best learned (see Chapters 3, 7, 10, and 11). Listening skills develop more readily through participation in real-life activities than in exercises. If a child repeats "May I have some more, please?" as part of a training exercise, his teacher might reward him with a pat on the back. If he repeats the same thing in a real-life situation—at the table—he is likely to receive a second helping, which is far more rewarding!

A child's ability to receive a message through hearing is not dependent upon his capacity to discriminate and identify *all* of its component sounds, but on his skill in obtaining *sufficient* cues to understand its meaning. The ways in which speech patterns vary with meaning are the child's guide in his acquisition of a cue system that permits him to decode speech signals. It is through the child's search for meaning—through his struggle to determine the speaker's intent—that he comes to realize what acoustic cues are significant. At first, his cue system may consist of a few grossly different patterns. As he succeeds in understanding more and more of what is said, he will automatically make finer and finer discriminations and come to identify some speech patterns categorically. His ultimate achievements in this respect will, of course, depend upon the nature and extent of his hearing impairment. Our view, then, is that the majority of hearing-impaired children, given hearing aids that provide them with optimal gain for the detection of sound and adequate practice in arriving at the meaning of spoken language, will learn most of the auditory discrimination and identification skills that are possible for them, without formal training on discrimination tasks.

Formal training must, of course, be provided for those who do not develop ability to discriminate and to identify sounds spontaneously and for those for whom even the best personal hearing aids are inadequate. Many personal hearing aids do not, for example, amplify fricative sounds as well as the larger, hard-wire systems which employ free-standing microphones, and headphones. Practice in the discrimination and production of fricative sounds may therefore be better given on such systems. Following such practice, the child may be able to make these discriminations using the reduced cues provided through his own hearing aid. We do not, therefore, recommend that auditory training be abandoned. Rather, we recommend that such training be viewed as a supplement to auditory experience and as an integral part of language and speech training.

Auditory Management

Auditory management of a hearing-impaired child may be viewed as the process of ensuring optimal use of residual hearing in his acquisition of the skills involved in communicating through spoken language. We have stated (above) that these skills are best learned in real-life situations from the earliest months of life. Auditory management of the child therefore involves manipulation of such situations so that the child can benefit fully from them. Placing the emphasis on learning informally through experience rather than formally through training, does not mean leaving the child to sink or swim in an unstructured sea of spoken language. Informal situations can be structured, and the more severe the child's hearing impairment, the more structured situations must be if he is to learn.

The first requirement in structuring situations for a hearing-impaired child is to ensure that he can detect noise-free speech at optimal listening levels. To meet this requirement, the child must

(a) have carefully selected and well-fitted hearing aids, and

(b) hear his own and others' speech at levels well in excess of background noise. We have discussed the fitting and selection of hearing aids in Chapter 6. We shall discuss speech/noise ratios later.

The second requirement in structuring situations is to ensure that the child's comprehension of speech is developed through the provision of abundant, meaningful, spoken language patterns—vocabulary and language, with which he can communicate his interests and feelings, discuss his ongoing activities, and express his needs. This is not as hard to achieve as it sounds. Before school, for example, one can talk and ask about clothes while dressing, food while eating or preparing meals, parts of the body while bathing, pain following a fall, or joy during a pleasant experience. Any novel or routine activity will serve. At school, countless situations and activities, related to academic work or not, can be devised and similarly exploited by a creative teacher/clinician.

The third requirement is to evaluate progress along the three dimensions which reflect the child's use of residual hearing, namely:

(a) speech reception,

(b) speech production, and

(c) spoken language.

Working informally to develop language should not be a hit-

or-miss affair (see Chapter 11). Informality does not mean that one is able to discard measures of progress. Systematic observation and testing are essential if an informal approach is to be successful. In order to know what to teach, one must know what a child has learned or failed to learn, what he has retained or failed to retain, and what skills he should develop next. One must also observe and evaluate, in order to determine whether the child's hearing aids are adequate under the conditions in which they are used, and whether supplementary training or special-purpose instruments should be used to spur achievement.

Speech Detection and Hearing Impairment

Particular patterns of speech can be detected only if (1) hearing is present over the frequency range in which they occur, and if (2) the patterns are of sufficient intensity to reach or exceed the child's threshold. Knowledge of the acoustic properties of speech and of the child's thresholds (see Chapter 4) allows one to predict with considerable accuracy whether or not particular sounds will be audible to the child. The following discussion illustrates this statement with reference to the curves plotted in Figure 7.1.

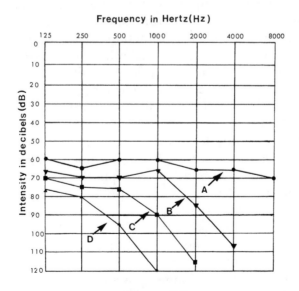

Figure 7.1
Audiograms of four hypothetical children (see text for discussion).

The child whose audiogram is shown as curve A in Figure 7.1 can be expected, given appropriate amplification, to detect all sounds of speech, since hearing is present over the complete speech frequency range (80–8000 Hz). The child whose audiogram is shown as curve B could also be expected to detect all speech sounds, but to miss some of the components of the fricatives and the high-frequency bursts of plosives. The [s], for example, has two main formants, one around 3000 Hz and the other just under 8000 Hz. Since, for child B, hearing is present at 3000 Hz and absent at 8000 Hz, he will not detect the total energy of this sound. In isolation, it will therefore be less audible to him than to a child with audiometric curve A. In effect, it may be detected at about 10 yards by the one child A, and only at about 10 inches by child B, given that both have appropriate hearing aids. Since child B will normally be within 10 inches of the microphone of his hearing aid, he may be expected to detect his own production of [s] but not to detect it consistently in the speech of others. Of course, since there are variant cues (consonant-to-vowel and vowel-to-consonant transitions) to the presence of [s] produced in context, a child with the hearing levels depicted as curve B should be able to detect the presence of [s] in running speech once he knows what cues to listen for. He may learn to listen for such cues spontaneously, or he may require specific training. If carried out as part of a speech teaching program, such training would increase the child's awareness of the production of the sound in syllables, words, and sentences by himself and others. Carried out as part of language training, it would increase the child's awareness of the [s] in various contexts, but particularly as a marker for plurals (hat/hats), possessives (John/John's) and third person singular verbs (walk/walks).

The important thing for children with hearing levels shown as curves A and B in Figure 7.1 is not so much what sounds they cannot detect, but the abundance of speech patterns that should be audible to them if they use appropriate hearing aids. All prosodic features of speech (intonation, duration, stress, etc.) can usually be detected by such children, as can all vowels, all voiced consonants, and most variant cues on manner, place, and voicing (see Chapter 4). Children with such hearing levels should learn most of their speech and language naturally and spontaneously through audition.

Children with hearing levels approximating curve C in Figure

7.1 should be able to detect all prosodic features of speech, and the low-frequency components of all vowels and some consonants. Generally, cues on manner of consonant production and the presence of voicing can be detected with such residual hearing. Few acoustic cues on place of consonant production would be detected because place cues lie almost exclusively between 1500 and 3500 Hz. Fricatives other than [ʃ], and the burst energy of plosives, would also be inaudible. Children with such hearing levels can usually acquire good control of voice patterns, develop natural sounding vowels, and approximate many words if they begin wearing hearing aids in the first year or so of life. Because so much of the acoustic information in speech cannot be detected through audition if there is no hearing above 1500 Hz, speech-reading skills must be developed to supplement the available residual audition of children having similar audiometric curves.

Hearing of the type depicted as curve D in Figure 7.1 constitutes a profound barrier to the acquisition of speech. With appropriate amplification, children with such hearing impairment can detect the first formants of most vowels, and hence most of the prosodic patterns of speech should also be audible. Because the frequency range in such cases is extremely limited, only those acoustic cues on consonants supplied by time and intensity changes can usually be detected by such children. In these cases, speechreading is usually the primary avenue of verbal learning, with hearing serving only as a supplementary modality.

In certain cases, left-hand corner audiograms represent a tactile rather than an auditory response. Children with such audiograms may feel, rather than hear, tonal stimuli. Alternatively, tactile and auditory responses may both be present. It is difficult to differentiate low-frequency tactile from auditory responses, except by advanced audiological tests. The main feature differentiating the two types of response is the ability to discriminate small differences in pitch. Touch is inferior to hearing in this respect. Before the child is able to respond to advanced testing, tactile responses may be suspected if he fails to develop controlled pitch variation in his voice in spite of efficient training. However, since a child's control of the pitch of his voice is often a reflection on inadequate auditory stimulation and ineffective speech training, conclusions regarding such thresholds in young children are hard to reach. Even if low-frequency thresholds may be tactile rather than auditory in origin, amplification which permits sound to reach these thresholds is to be recommended; the tactile sensations thus provided can significantly supplement information gained through speechreading.

There are certain dangers inherent in the attempt to predict the detection of a sound by a child on the basis of his audiogram. If the audiogram is unreliable, then the predictions made will be equally so. If the child has residual hearing which lies beyond the upper limits of the audiometer, but within reach of a hearing aid, then the predictions will underestimate the range of sounds the child can detect. No test of aided speech detection can be more accurate than one which employs speech stimuli presented to the child through his hearing aids.

Aided Audiograms

Aided audiograms are produced by plotting the child's threshold to tones presented as the child is wearing his hearing aid. The curve that results—when compared with the child's regular (unaided) audiogram—indicates approximately how much gain the hearing aid provides at each frequency tested. Thus, if the child's unaided threshold at 1000 Hz is 90 dB and the child's aided threshold at this frequency is 40 dB, then one knows that the gain provided by the hearing aid at that frequency is about $90 - 40 = 50$ dB. If one increased or decreased the gain of the hearing aid by changing its volume control setting, the aided threshold would reflect that change. Aided audiograms therefore show how well or poorly a hearing aid helps a child to detect sound. It cannot be used as a measure of how well or poorly a child uses his residual hearing, since such a measure would demand tests involving discrimination, identification, and comprehension of speech.

Aided audiograms may allow one to demonstrate that a child has hearing beyond the limits of the audiometer. Thus a child may not respond at 2000 Hz when tested with an audiometer which can produce no more than 110 dB, yet can respond at this frequency when aided. Such a case is illustrated by Figure 7.2. In this case, the hearing aid was known to provide 55 dB gain at 2000 Hz. Since the child responded at 60 dB in the aided condition we know that the child's threshold for 2000 Hz must lie at about $60 + 55 = 115$ dB.

Aided thresholds can be predicted to within a few decibels if the child's unaided thresholds and the gain of the aid are known. The

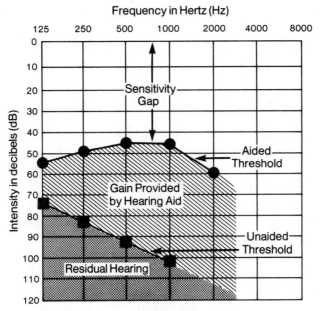

Figure 7.2

An audiogram showing both aided and unaided thresholds for a hypothetical child. The difference between the two thresholds is a measure of the gain provided by the hearing aid. The fact that hearing aids cannot compensate fully for severe or profound hearing impairment is indicated by the sensitivity gap at the top of the chart. Sounds of less than 45–50 dB would be inaudible to a child with aided thresholds as shown. Some children's sensitivity gaps might be reduced if they could tolerate more powerful hearing aids, but such is not always the case (see text).

prediction will not be exact for several reasons: (1) Aided thresholds are measured in a free-field—through loud-speakers—whereas unaided thresholds are usually measured through headphones. There are usually differences in thresholds measured under the two conditions. (2) The stimuli used for testing under the two conditions may be different. Steady-state pure tones of the type usually presented through headphones cannot be used reliably in a free-field because they often cause standing waves (changes in intensity due to reflection of the sound from walls or other objects in the sound field). Tones that change in frequency (warble) must therefore be used in free-field testing. (3) Even if the above variables were controlled, the hearing aid's response, as measured on standard equipment, may be modified by the child's earmold (see below). (4) The child's size and position in the sound field relative to the loudspeakers can influence the intensity of the sound reaching the hearing aid. Predictions based on hearing aid specifications and comparisons of unaided and aided thresholds are therefore imprecise and must be made with caution.

Hearing Aids and Auditory Sensitivity

That hearing aids fail to compensate for hearing impairment is best illustrated through further reference to Figure 7.2. The aided audiogram depicted in this figure shows that the particular hearing aid used in this case has left what we describe as a "sensitivity gap" of about 50 dB. The hearing aid only partially compensated for this child's profound hearing impairment. It did not restore hearing sensitivity to normal levels. Had it done so, the child's aided thresholds would have been at or near audiometric zero. It is rarely either possible or desirable to provide a severely or profoundly hearing-impaired child with a hearing aid that has a gain equivalent at all frequencies to his hearing impairment. Hearing aids with such gain, even if they could be manufactured, would tend to amplify sounds either so that acoustic feedback would be unavoidable, or so that speech and noise would become uncomfortably loud. Most severely and profoundly hearing-impaired children therefore have a significant sensitivity gap. It is unusual for the sensitivity gap of children with unaided thresholds, as shown in Figure 7.2, to be less than 40 dB.

Acoustics and Auditory Sensitivity

Much can be done to help a child compensate for a sensitivity gap and thus receive speech more effectively. For example, one can optimize the clarity of the auditory signal, let the child speech-read, use tactile cues, or all three. The first possibility, rendering the auditory signal optimal, is the one that we shall discuss here.

Optimal clarity of speech depends on several factors: the speaker's articulation, the intensity at which it reaches the listener, and the extent to which it is mixed with noise. Let us assume that speech is articulated well and produced at average levels of intensity. The intensity at which speech reaches the listener will then depend mainly on distance. Within limits, its overall level will fall by approximately 6 dB every time distance is doubled. Thus, if at about three inches from the mouth it were 80 dB (HL), at six inches it would be 74 dB; at one foot, 68 dB; at two feet, 62 dB; at four feet, 56 dB; at 8 feet, 50 dB and so on. Now, reference to Figure 7.2 shows that at distances of eight feet or more with the particular hearing aid provided, the child would be unable to detect all speech sounds. Thus, to compensate for a sensitivity gap, one's first step would be to determine the distance at which speech sounds are audible to the child, and always to talk to him well within that distance.

Sound is reflected from hard surfaces in much the same way that light is reflected by a mirror. In normal surroundings, reflection of the speech signal from walls, ceilings, floors, and furniture will contribute to its overall intensity. At distances of about eight feet or more, the intensity contributed by reflected sound in a room may amount to several decibels. In real-life situations, doubling distance beyond eight feet will therefore result in less than a 6 dB drop in intensity but a substantial decrease in clarity.

In addition to reflecting speech, hard surfaces will help to cause and reflect noise. As one moves over an uncovered floor, contact between one's shoes and the floor creates sound which is then reflected to and from the floor and other hard surfaces. Such noise can substantially reduce the clarity of speech. Carpeting helps to prevent both the creation of noise and its reflection. Other soft furnishings also absorb rather than reflect sound. It is therefore better to work and play with hearing-impaired children in surroundings which prevent and absorb noise, since such surroundings enhance the clarity of the speech signal. In playrooms and nursery schools, carpets and draperies should be routine furnishing. If necessary, acoustic tiles should be placed on ceilings and walls to prevent undue reverberation of sound. A piece of cloth or carpet on the table used for play activities in a nursery can make the difference between the child learning to hear speech and learning to ignore sound.

The number of decibels by which speech is more intense than noise is called the speech-to-noise (or signal-to-noise) ratio. A speech/noise ratio of 30 dB permits the quietest sounds of speech to be heard without interference by noise. As the speech/noise ratio decreases, more and more of the speech signal becomes masked by noise and thus is less intelligible. Children who are learning their mother tongue, and adults who are learning a second language, require greater speech intensities and greater speech/noise ratios than skilled listeners in order to understand what is said. The single most effective technique is to speak at normal levels close to the listener. Shouting does not help hearing-impaired people because it raises the level of voiced sounds, (which they can usually hear fairly well), without substantially increasing the level of unvoiced consonants, which are usually less audible.

Room acoustics can play a major role in determining whether or not a child can learn through the use of residual audition. It makes little sense to spend hundreds of dollars every few years on hearing aids, and thousands of dollars annually on a child's education if the acoustic conditions—which can be optimized for a relatively small sum—prevent the hearing aids and the teacher/clinician from working effectively.

Special-Purpose Hearing Aids

Three types of special-purpose amplification systems are commonly used in the habilitative treatment of hearing-impaired children. These are hard-wire systems (group hearing aids and speech training aids), loop induction systems, and radio systems. All three have two things in common: They reproduce sound without significant decrease in intensity over distance, and they permit speech/noise ratios that are superior to those usually obtained with individual hearing aids.

Hard-wire Systems

Hard-wire amplification systems are those in which the microphones and the headphones are separately connected to the amplifier by means of electric cables. The simplest form of such a system is the individual speech training aid which has one microphone, one amplifier, and one pair of headphones. The most complex form of such a system is the group hearing aid, in which several of these components are interconnected in such a way that amplification can be provided for a large class of children. These aids reproduce speech with high fidelity and at levels of intensity that can be precisely controlled by the teacher/clinician and/or child. Because the microphone(s) in such systems can be held or worn close to the mouth of the speaker, speech patterns can be transmitted at levels well above those of background noise. Such systems can therefore be used effectively in relatively poor acoustic environments.

Hard-wire systems which employ high-quality headphones can provide amplification up to or even beyond 8000 Hz. Thus, they are capable of reproducing a wider range of frequencies than individual hearing aids, few of which currently provide significant amplification beyond 3500 Hz. Children who have residual hearing for high frequencies can therefore often detect components of sounds (such as [s], for example) that might be inaudible to them through their personal hearing aids.

There is some controversy over the use of hard-wire systems as a supplement to the use of personal hearing aids. It has been argued that two different patterns of sound are presented if two forms of amplification are used, and that this would be confusing to the child. It is claimed that the exclusive use of personal hearing aids ensures that speech heard by the child has a consistent quality. We do not support these arguments. As shown above, speech quality changes with speaker, with distance from the speaker, with the speech/noise ratio, among other variables. Thus, speech signals are not consistent. Exposure to speech amplified by a hard-wire system can often help children to detect sound, and differences between sounds, that might not be audible through their personal aids. Awareness of the more complete pattern that a hard-wire system can provide cannot possibly detract from perception of the partial pattern received through a child's own hearing aids at other times. To suggest otherwise would be akin to saying that the child's perception of an elephant's trunk is diminished rather than enhanced by occasionally seeing it attached to the whole animal.

Of course, some children can hear sufficient cues to learn speech and language spontaneously through audition with their personal hearing aids; others can not. For those who can not, hard-wire systems may help by providing acoustic cues that are not otherwise available. The value of hard-wire systems for such children is most readily seen in the teaching of speech. Such systems can often provide the extra information a child needs in order to differentiate one sound from another—[s] from [ʃ], for example, or [k] from [t]. Once the child has learned such acoustic distinctions, he can more readily imitate these sounds. As he hears and produces them correctly using the hard-wire system, he will build the orosensory and motor images that will enable him to produce the sound through feedforward rather than feedback processes (see Chapter 8). He will therefore be able to produce

sounds that he would not have acquired had his auditory experience been limited just to listening through personal hearing aids.
Children's speech largely reflects what they hear. We know of
relatively few severely and profoundly hearing-impaired children
whose speech indicates that their personal hearing aids fully meet
their needs.

There are disadvantages to hard-wire systems. The principal
problem is that they tether a child to positions within the radius of
the cord leading from the amplifier to his headphones, and thus
restrict the type of learning activity that can be pursued. Creative
teacher/clinicians should, however, have few problems in devising
suitable, lively learning situations for short periods, if the child
needs to be trained on a hard-wire system. A second possible
problem is that headphones worn for more than brief periods
may prove to be uncomfortable for some young children. Discomfort is often claimed by children whose interest is not sufficiently
engaged. The problem is best solved by keeping activities short
and interesting, or finding more comfortable types of earphone
cushion.

Loop Induction Systems

Telephone receivers create a small electromagnetic field as they
reproduce the speech of the caller. If a small coil of wire is placed
against the receiver—in this electromagnetic field—the energy
present will induce current to flow through the coil. The pattern
of current that flows through the coil will be exactly the same as
that created by the caller as he speaks into his telephone. Sound
can thus be transmitted by using an amplification system driven
by a coil rather than by a microphone. Hearing aids that allow one
to listen to a telephone call by switching from the microphone (M)
to a *telecoil* (T) are in common use. Hearing aids that allow one to
use the microphone and the telecoil (M + T) simultaneously are
also available. These should always be used with children, since
they need to hear their own speech as well as that of others.

Hearing aids that contain telecoils can also be used with loop
induction systems. These systems are created by connecting a loop
of wire that circles a given area—a room, a hall, an arena—to an
amplifier or hi-fi set. Speech amplified by such equipment causes
current to flow through the loop of wire and to create an electromagnetic field over the entire area surrounded by the wire
loop. Using a hearing aid equipped with a telecoil, a child can

receive speech at the same level of intensity anywhere within the loop. Thus a teacher/clinician talking into her microphone at one end of a room is heard as if she is talking directly into the child's hearing aid even though he may be at the far end of the room. Consequently, the teacher's speech will be heard at levels well above existing room noise. The great advantage of loop induction over hard-wire systems in homes and classrooms is that the child's movement is not restricted. The disadvantage of loop induction systems is that they cannot be used in adjacent classrooms because the electromagnetic field of a loop extends outside the looped area, creating a condition known as *overspill*.

Overspill leads to a lesson in one classroom being heard by children in another. Loop induction systems can be used most effectively under conditions in which overspill is of no concern. For example, a loop system can be installed in a child's home. Unless there are neighbors who also use a loop system, it does not matter that the loop's electromagnetic field extends beyond the looped area. In fact, it may be an advantage for the child to be able to hear clearly upstairs, downstairs, or outside on the lawn. Similarly, such a system can be employed in a single class of a neighborhood school, around a tennis court, or in a church. The loop of wire is simply passed around the area, under the carpet, fixed to the walls, or suspended from the ceiling. When used under any of these conditions—and many more—loop induction systems allow speech to reach the child at high levels of intensity and at good speech/noise ratios.

Loop induction systems are easy to construct—even for the amateur. Such a system requires a good quality microphone, a moderately powerful (5 to 10 watt) amplifier, and a length of wire. Most hi-fi stereo sets can be used both for their normal purpose and as amplifiers for a loop induction system. In such an ar-rangement, the ends of the loop are connected to the terminals provided for one of the loudspeakers. Either a radio microphone/transmitter can be used to drive the system, or a reg-ular microphone can be plugged in. It is essential that the loop of wire, which replaces an 8-ohm speaker, has 8 ohms of resistance. This resistance is provided by 400 feet of 23-gauge wire, or 800 feet of 20-gauge wire. To make the loop one merely has to meas-ure around the selected area, wind the appropriate length of wire around it, and connect each of the ends to loudspeaker terminals.

We have found that parents of severely or profoundly hearing-impaired children can often provide better auditory experience for them using loop induction than using the microphone system of the hearing aids. For example, when the toddler is at the stage of following mother around the house while she makes the beds, dusts the furniture, prepares a meal, and so on, she can provide a running commentary on everything that she does. With a radio microphone worn around her neck, she can be sure that (1) her speech will not be masked by any of the sounds she makes as she works, and that (2) the child will receive her speech clearly even when the distance between them might preclude the child from hearing her through just the microphone of his hearing aid. Of course, under most conditions the telecoil and the microphone should be in simultaneous use so that the child can also hear his own speech.

There are certain occasions, however, when listening through loop induction alone is more advantageous than listening through both microphone and telecoil. For example, while watching a movie, with the projector in the same room, the mechanical noise it makes can drastically interfere with the child's reception of the sound track. If the amplifier of the projector is used to drive an induction loop, the hearing aid can be switched to telecoil (T), and mechanical noise completely excluded. A similar advantage can be obtained if a television set is used to drive an induction loop. Not only can room noise be excluded by listening only via the induction loop, but distortions inevitably introduced by the loudspeaker of the television set and the microphone of the hearing aid can thus be bypassed.

Small induction loops create smaller electromagnetic fields than large induction loops. Thus, to prevent overspill into an adjacent room, an induction loop can be wound under a chair or a table. Induction loops with coils no larger than a fingernail can even be constructed. When held or attached (by means of Velcro, for example) to the outer casing of a hearing aid switched to the telecoil, they can create listening conditions equal to those provided by a much larger induction loop. The miniature receiver provided with most television sets and transistor radios contains a coil that makes an ideal "miniloop." One can simply remove the diaphragm of a miniature receiver to prevent it reproducing audible sound, and cover the exposed coil with any non-metallic material. The coil, already housed in a casing and attached to a long cord, becomes a miniloop when plugged into a television set, radio, or another amplifying device. Placed on or near the casing of a hearing aid switched to the T position, it can substantially enhance the speech signal received, relative to that provided through the microphone.* A miniloop used with a radio or television set normally cuts out the loudspeaker, and thus permits the child (or an older hearing aid user) to listen to programs without them being heard by others. This arrangement is often desirable. Both the loop and the loudspeaker can be used at the same time if a small modification, which can be made by any competent technician, is made to the output system of the television or radio set.

Radio Hearing Aids

Hearing aids that provide input from a radio microphone/transmitter worn by the teacher/clinician or the parent are now in common use. The most popular forms of radio hearing aids are those that function both as regular hearing aids and as pre-tuned radio receivers. They permit the child to hear his own voice through the microphone contained in the instrument, and that of the teacher/clinician or parent through the radio circuit. Interchangeable modules (crystals) allow the child's receiver to be pre-tuned to one of several wave lengths. This arrangement allows a number of microphone-transmitters to be used simultaneously in one area. Thus two or more teacher/clinicians, transmitting on different wave lengths, can work with two or more groups of children in the same class at the same time without interference.

Radio hearing aids have two main advantages over hard-wire and loop induction systems. First, they require no installation. They can therefore be used inside or outside the home or classroom, or in several different classrooms, on the same day. Second, unlike other systems (including regular hearing aids), they can operate over a range of several hundred feet, extending a child's auditory experience in many ways. For example, they can permit communication over a distance during excursions to places of interest such as a zoo or a farm; they can be used for coaching in sports such as skiing, where the instructor would often be too far

---

*Construction of this form of "miniloop" was first demonstrated to the writers by Mr. Charles Munro of the Montreal Oral School for the Deaf.

away to be heard with a regular hearing aid; and they can permit severely and profoundly hearing-impaired children to function more adequately in special or regular schools as they move from one classroom to another during the day. Thus the area over which a child can be active and yet remain in auditory contact is quite large.

Radio aids have some disadvantages compared to other systems. They are much more expensive than regular hearing aids and loop-induction systems. They have lower fidelity than hard-wire systems. They are much larger than regular hearing aids and are therefore more awkward for children—particularly young children—to wear. Like loop induction systems, radio aids provide the same amplified signal to both ears. In this respect they are inferior to binaural hearing aids.

Our discussion of special-purpose hearing aids indicates that we consider them necessary for some children on some occasions. Certainly, there are hearing-impaired children who can manage to acquire natural speech and language skills spontaneously without ever having to use them. However, the more severely hearing-impaired the child, the more likely it is that one or more forms of special-purpose aid can be used with him to advantage. The decision as to whether or not to use a special-purpose system should be based on only one consideration: namely, whether it can help the child detect speech more adequately than his personal hearing aids alone. In many learning situations—speech lessons, language instruction, participation in class at a distance from the teacher—the use of one or more of these systems might well permit the child to receive more complete speech patterns at better speech/noise ratios than would otherwise be the case. Optimal detection is a necessary condition for optimal discrimination, identification, and comprehension of speech. One should not, therefore, reject the use of special-purpose aids without careful consideration of what they can offer a particular child. This is true particularly in the early stages of training, when the child's restricted knowledge of speech and language severely limits the cues as to meaning that might otherwise be derived from verbal context.

Auditory Experience and Auditory Training

The quantity and content of the auditory-verbal experience

provided for a child significantly influence his ability to use whatever residual hearing he may possess. The quantity of auditory-
verbal experience that a child receives is determined by two
things: how well he can detect the speech signal, and the extent to
which he is exposed to spoken language communication. All the
care lavished upon the child's acoustic management—his audiological assessment, his hearing aids, and his acoustic
environment—is wasted unless one talks with the child, has others
talk with him, and ensures that an abundance of speech communication takes place within the child's auditory range. Such
observations may appear self-evident, yet we have found that
some parents have great difficulty in finding things to say to their
hearing-impaired child, and cannot easily encourage other members of the family to relate to him through speech communication.
We also know teachers who are so concerned with the children's
academic skills that they make minimal auditory-verbal contact
with them. There are also many residential schools where
auditory-verbal experience simply cannot be gained in out-of-
class hours. Normally hearing children can acquire much of their
auditory-verbal experience indirectly and at a considerable distance from speakers. In contrast, most hearing-impaired children
have but a limited auditory range, and must be spoken to directly
if they are to learn verbally.

• The content of auditory-verbal experience provided for a child
is appropriate only if he can derive meaning from what is said. At
the most elementary level, some meaning can be derived without
understanding of words—from the speaker's tone of voice, along
with nonverbal cues provided through other sense modalities and
situational context. Even animals can derive meaning from
spoken language at this level—e.g., a dog will fetch his master's
slippers when commanded to do so only if the tone of voice is
right and the situation is familiar. At the most advanced level,
meaning is derived through ability to interpret complex sentences
in which subtle nuances are conveyed almost entirely by the apt
choice of words. Most children's ability to derive meaning from
what is said lies somewhere between these two extremes.

Progress from the most elementary to the most advanced level
of auditory-verbal comprehension occurs as the child becomes
able to understand more and more words, and acquires an increasing number of linguistic rules. At the same time, such progress is marked by the child's decreasing reliance upon nonverbal

cues. Comprehension of auditory-verbal material is therefore best fostered by ensuring that the child receives meaningful auditory patterns in regularly occurring situations until they become familiar, and that nonverbal and situational cues are gradually reduced. This principle applies at any stage in a child's development, however restricted residual hearing may be.

The rate at which a child learns to comprehend auditory-verbal material will depend upon several factors, including:

a) the extent to which the hearing aid compensates for his hearing impairment,

b) his intelligence,

c) the parents' skills,

d) the teacher/clinician's skills,

e) the suitability and complexity of the auditory-verbal material, and

f) the consistency and frequency with which this material is presented.

A child's failure to learn certain auditory patterns, or to learn them quickly, is often due not to the hearing impairment, but to the use of inappropriate auditory-verbal patterns. To be appropriate they must be meaningful (relate to the child's interests and needs), and they must either consolidate or extend his understanding and use of spoken language. To select language forms that fit the child's requirements, one must know the child as an active being, and his current level of linguistic achievement. If the child is unable to learn to understand and to use particular speech patterns through hearing—and if there is no doubt that they have been selected and presented with sufficient skill and often enough to ensure their familiarity—then another sense modality must be employed without undue delay.

Just as auditory-verbal experience should relate closely to language development, so should auditory training be closely allied to speech acquisition. Traditional auditory training programs typically begin with discrimination of nonverbal sounds. There may be some fun and some merit in training a child to distinguish between a horn, a bell, a drum, and a whistle, but one can expect little or no improvement in auditory speech reception to result from such training. If one's aim is to develop speech reception skills through the use of residual audition, then the presentation of speech rather than nonverbal patterns should be required, for the following reasons: speech segments are of much shorter duration than such nonverbal sounds; the two types of sounds are processed in different hemispheres of the brain; speech patterns provide a greater range of contrast and similarity; training involving speech is a direct approach; and more precise and more durable auditory discrimination and identification skills will result when the child's speech system is employed as part of the listening process, since auditory-vocal feedback skills are also developed.

The concepts presented in this chapter differ greatly from those that were current when hearing aids were first developed. The emphasis was then upon auditory training, whereas present-day work is more strongly focused upon auditory experience related to each child's abilities, needs, and activities. Further discussion of the use of residual hearing is contained in Chapters 9, 10, and 11, which are concerned with the development of speech and language skills.

ANNOTATED BIBLIOGRAPHY

Griffiths, C. (Ed.)   *Proceedings of the International Conference on Auditory Techniques.* Springfield, Ill.: Charles C Thomas, 1974.

This is, as the title indicates, a collection of papers delivered at a conference. Although the book does not provide a comprehensive coverage of aural habilitation, it does include a variety of interesting and worthwhile chapters by numerous people who are world leaders in the application of modern technology in the education of hearing-impaired children. Most papers are easy to read, but few provide references to other material.

Pollack, D.   *Educational Audiology for the Limited Hearing Infant.* Springfield, Ill.: Charles C Thomas, 1970.

This book was written by a highly experienced teacher/clinician whose work with hearing-impaired children derived from the most advanced thought and practice that evolved in Europe following World War II. It describes a practical system for maximizing the use of residual hearing in the education of young children, one that closely parallels the type of work that is advocated by the authors of the present text.

Ross, M.   *Principles of Aural Rehabilitation*. Indianapolis: The Bobbs Merrill Co., 1972.
The various factors underlying successful rehabilitation are briefly described in this text, which is written at an introductory level. Emphasis is placed upon the need for early use of amplification.

Ross, M., and Giolas, T. G. (Eds.)   *Auditory Management of the Hearing-Impaired Child*. Baltimore, Md.: University Park Press, 1978.
A compilation of papers prepared for in-depth discussion at a small, select conference, this text is the most comprehensive treatment of the use of residual audition published to date. All contributors are internationally known and respected. Their frank discussion of other participants' papers and the care taken by the editors to make the text cohesive renders the book easy to use and the most valuable source of information on the use of hearing that has ever been available.

Sanders, D. A.   *Aural Rehabilitation*. Englewood Cliffs, N.J.: Prentice-Hall, 1971.
A classic in the field of audiology, this book presents a theoretical framework within which the nature of problems arising from hearing impairment is examined. Some aspects of the book are now outdated—e.g., the standards relating to hearing aid measurement have been changed—but most of the text is still ahead of current practice in the field and all of it is well worth reading.

8. Vision and Touch in Speech Reception and Speech Production

*W*hen people speak, they expect others to listen. It is taken for granted that speech is an acoustic event perceived through hearing. Speech is also an articulatory activity and, under some circumstances, watching the speaker form words helps the listener to understand what is said. Vision helps most where background noise is present and least in quiet situations. In speech reception by normally hearing listeners, then, two senses are used: audition, which is predominant, and vision, which is sometimes used to supplement audition.

Of course, speech reception is an activity that involves the brain even more than the ears and the eyes. In receiving a spoken message, one is searching for the underlying meaning of what is said. How easily one grasps the meaning of a message depends not only upon how clearly it is spoken, but upon how familiar one is with the topic, the vocabulary used, the grammar of the language, and so on. This being so, one can often understand a spoken message which is incomplete, just as one can decipher a postcard in which some words are illegible. For example, most people would be able to supply the last word in the sentence, "Mommy's baking a _____ ."

One's senses are employed somewhat differently in speech production than in speech reception (see Figure 8.1). Speakers use their hearing to monitor what they say, but unless they use a mirror, they cannot see their own speech movements. However, at either a conscious or unconscious level, they can feel where the tongue makes contact with various points in the vocal tract (touch)

133

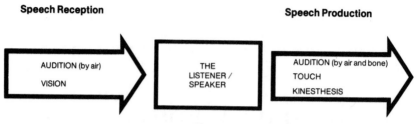

Figure 8.1

A schematic diagram of the senses as they are used in speech reception and speech production. In speech production one receives direct feedback through three modalities, as compared with two in speech reception.

and how the speech organs move (kinesthesis). The auditory patterns of speech received by a speaker differ from those received by a listener. When others speak, the sound waves created are air-borne and enter the listener's auditory system via the ear canal. When speakers hear themselves, they receive both air-conducted and bone-conducted sound. Their own speech reaches them both through the ear canal and through the vibration of the skull. This is why people do not know how they sound to others until they hear a good quality tape recording of their own speech.

Feedback and Feedforward

The skilled speaker makes less use of his senses to monitor what he says than the child who is learning to talk. Once spoken language skills have been mastered, it is possible to speak intelligibly without using hearing at all. Thus, people who become totally deaf from meningitis after they have well-established speech skills continue to be able to talk, although some phonemes, such as /s/, may eventually become distorted. Similarly, sensation in the mouth may be blocked by an anesthetic, yet the normal speaker can make himself understood even when his speech organs are numb. Most people who have had dental treatment know this from personal experience. These examples demonstrate that, although speakers usually employ hearing, touch, and kinesthesis to obtain feedback, factors other than feedback govern speech production in skilled talkers.

Feedback provides the speaker with knowledge of correctness—whether he has said what he intended to say. He may receive feedback directly from his senses, from his listeners, or from both. He may hear or feel that he said "the right wag" instead of "the white rag." On the other hand, he may only become aware of his mistake through the listeners' reactions. This example illustrates an important point: namely, that a speaker receives feedback only *after* he has produced a series of sounds. It does not assist him in producing the series of sounds correctly in the first place.

Correct production of a series of sounds—a word or a sentence—is governed by a feedforward process. Feedforward is the chain of unconscious activities that precedes the expression of an idea: the formulation of the thought in words, the transmission of correctly sequenced commands from the brain to the speech organs, and the coordination of the movements of these organs. Because the task is so complex, it cannot be carried out smoothly unless all of the activities involved have been practiced until they are automatic. It is during early infancy—in episodes of vocalization, babbling, verbal play, and repetitive speech—that feedback plays its most important role. It is on the basis of information provided by sensory feedback during such activities that the child can practice sound sequences to automaticity and develop feedforward skills.

Vision

The extent to which vision is used in speech reception by normally hearing children is unknown. Babies can imitate visible mouth movements when they are only a few months old. Many of the first words produced by children—for example, "up," "bye bye," and "mummy"—contain sounds that are relatively easy to see on the lips. School-age children tend to watch their teachers intently (when they are paying attention) and may thus be using vision to help them follow speech in the noisy conditions that typically prevail in classrooms. Certainly, young children who are asked "What sound am I making?" when a vowel is silently formed on the lips will usually respond correctly. Such observations imply that most normally hearing children have basic speechreading skills, at the least.

Speechreading

Speechreading is much more important to hearing-impaired children than to their normally hearing peers. At best, however, speechreading is a very poor substitute for hearing because so many sounds look alike on the lips. For example, "pat," "bat," and "mat" are a group of words not readily distinguished by eye, as are "dot," "tot," and "not." The words "heat" and "eat" look alike on the lips because there are no visible components of the sound [h]. On account of many such problems, speechreading can only be effective as a supplement to hearing or if context supplies the child with the missing information.

When severely hearing-impaired children are given tests of simple word recognition, speechreading-plus-hearing typically yields an advantage of 15 to 20 percent over hearing alone. This is because speechreading helps the child to differentiate words that may sound alike to him, such as "bib," "bid," and "big." A common misconception is that a child who can score, say, 50 percent through speechreading alone and 50 percent through aided hearing alone will be able to score 100 percent using both audition and vision. This is not so, because some of the information received through one sense replicates that received through the other. For example, the child may recognize the vowel in a word like "feet" through both hearing and vision. An advantage of 15 to 20 percent for speechreading-plus-hearing over aided hearing alone may not appear to be very important. Such an advantage may, however, make the difference between the child being able to understand an everyday conversation and being completely unable to follow what is being said.

Of course, conversation is more than just a string of words. Running speech contains more cues on identity and meaning than isolated words. Situations provide cues. Thus, although "pike" and "bike" look alike on the lips, they are unlikely to be confused if the conversation takes place during a fishing trip or during a cycling tour. Similarly, cues are provided by context. If one has to speechread the words "half past two" when there has been no reference to time, the task is much harder than when these words are spoken in reply to questions like "What's the time?" or "When does the bus leave?" A knowledge of grammar also helps the speechreader. For children with a knowledge of grammar, the plural "boys" is unlikely to be mistaken for the singular "boy" if it occurs in the sentence "Two big boys helped me."

Speechreading is difficult on account of the partial and ambiguous information it provides, but it is by no means an impossible task. As with many other types of skills, children's ability to acquire competence in speechreading varies. Some totally deaf children do not become good speechreaders, while others learn their spoken language through speechreading and go on to obtain regular school diplomas and university degrees. The majority of hearing-impaired children have useful residual hearing, however, and hence are not called upon to learn through speechreading alone.

In order to learn how to speechread, children must have reasonably good eyesight. Failure is invited if the child has visual problems that are allowed to persist undetected or uncorrected. Sight should therefore be tested routinely.

Speechreading and Hearing

There is no question that totally deaf children must rely principally on speechreading in order to learn spoken language. There is also no question that speechreading should be only a supplement—never an alternative—to aided audition if the child has useful residual hearing. The only way to ensure that any residual audition present is used and developed as the primary receptive sense is to attempt to work first through audition. One should ensure that the most appropriate hearing aid is constantly worn, and employ vision only if the child consistently fails to respond through hearing. This does not imply that one should deprive the child of essential stimulation by spending years, months, or even weeks in a struggle to communicate with the child through an inadequate sense. Rather, one should present speech patterns several times over a period of days and observe the child carefully. If there is no response indicating that the child can hear when listening conditions are optimal, then the pattern should be presented visually. If the child then responds, one should try hearing again. One should conclude that the child needs to speechread a particular pattern only when he fails to react to further presentations of that pattern through audition. Children respond more readily to meaningful than to non-meaningful events, and auditory patterns that are not initially meaningful may become so. A child's failure to react to the first few presentations of a pattern is therefore inadequate as evidence that sound is inaudible. Further, because one speech pattern may be inaudible to a child, it must not be assumed that all speech patterns will be equally so (see Chapter 4).

Diagnosis of Speechreading Needs

Work with hearing-impaired children during infancy and into school life must be regarded as diagnostic in nature. An adequate diagnosis of needs cannot be made on the basis of clinical tests alone. Only through careful observation and the ongoing evaluation of a child's responses can it be decided whether he is totally deaf and therefore a candidate for a completely visual approach, whether his aided residual hearing should supplement speechreading, whether speechreading should supplement his aided hearing, or whether his potential when using a hearing aid is so good that speechreading should not be encouraged at all. Should aided residual hearing plus speechreaching prove to be inadequate for the spontaneous acquisition of spoken language skills, then carefully structured teaching to make speechreading effective must be provided. The principles underlying a structured approach are given below.

Speechreading Plus

Speechreading provides incomplete information as to what is said. To make speechreading effective, therefore, something else is needed to fill the gaps and resolve the ambiguities in the message received. The necessary additional information must be provided either by the child himself—through reference to stored knowledge and experience—or by the child using such reference together with additional cues provided by the speaker. What types of stored knowledge and experience can effectively supplement the speechread pattern? What additional cues can speakers provide? Brief answers to these questions are given below.

First, the child must become aware that speech communication is an important and meaningful activity, and that responses to speech have positive and direct advantages for him which affect his needs and happiness. To gain such knowledge, the child must be given abundant experience of speech in situations and activities that relate to his welfare and interests. Repetition of patterns in the recurring events of everyday life such as dressing, toilet, feeding, play, and so on, will then provide the required opportunities for him to derive meaning from the speechread form and, through familiarity and the process of association, acquire understanding of first words.

Second, the child should learn and store vocabulary relating to his experience. As an increasing number of visual word patterns are stored, the more readily will the child arrive at the meaning of the speech he sees, and the easier will it be for him to find new words adjacent to those that are already familiar. At the outset, the child does not know where one word ends and another begins in the continuous flow of speech. This is one reason why children take longer to learn first words than later words. This also applies to learning to receive speech through hearing. The task is harder through vision than through hearing, not only because certain speech sounds are invisible or can be confused with others, but because intonation and stress and rhythm—which help to define word boundaries—can be heard but not seen. This is not to imply that vocabulary should be taught through the use of single words. Such a procedure would inhibit the child's development of strategies to extract meaning and impede his development of language. Very little meaning or language resides in a single word.

Third, the child should develop speech skills. Even before he begins to comprehend speech, the child who has to rely upon speechreading should be encouraged to vocalize and be taught to speak as he acquires his initial vocabulary. Many teachers and parents fail to realize how much speech production can contribute to speech reception. Hence they may ignore speech development or excuse poor speech skills with statements such as, "Speech production is less important than language and understanding." Statements such as this are akin to saying "Peter is more important than his education." Just as education can enhance Peter's general development, so can speech provide skills that help vocabulary and language to grow.

If a child is taught how to produce differences between [p], [b] and [m], for example, he will realize that words which contain these sounds may look alike but are, in fact, different. His knowledge of words will be more precise than that of the child who cannot produce these different sounds. Further, the more clearly children talk, the more ready people are to enter into conversation with them. This in turn leads to more contacts that stimulate language growth. If begun early, the systematic development of speech takes relatively little time in a child's daily life. The alternatives are correction of faulty voice and word approximations that have become habitual by a later stage, and acceptance of permanently poor speech—which is not a necessary by-product of deafness. Correction in later childhood involves much more work than the initial development of good speech patterns. Furthermore, since other matters may be assigned higher priority, sufficient time may never be scheduled for speech training or correction in later school life.

Fourth, the child must acquire the rules that govern the use of language. Only when he has learned, stored and is able to use these rules will he be in a position to predict words and their order within sentences. For more detailed discussion of language and its role in perception, see Chapters 3, 10, and 11.

There are two types of additional cues that speakers can provide for speechreaders: those that clarify the intended meaning of the message, and those that help fill information gaps or reduce ambiguities in the message itself. Cues of the first type include relating what is said to the prevailing activity, ensuring that the context of the message is clear, checking that key words in the message are recognized, and using language structures that are familiar. Cues of the second type are provided by ensuring that residual hearing, hand cues, visual displays, or tactile aids (as the case may be) are used in such a way that sounds or differences between sounds that cannot be seen on the lips are conveyed to the child in some other way.

Visual Displays and Visual Cues

Many different types of visual displays and visual cues have been invented for the purpose of clarifying the nature of speech sounds that are inaudible to certain hearing-impaired children. Unfortunately their value has rarely been studied objectively and systematically. As a result, visual displays and visual cue systems have often been accepted on faith and used with children regardless of whether they need them or not, or rejected out of hand without adequate (or sometimes fair) evaluation. Since there are some hearing-impaired children who can benefit from visual supplements to speechreading, we shall briefly discuss apparent possibilities and limitations in their use. Prior to doing so, we wish to stress that no visual display or cue system can as effectively supplement speechreading as does residual hearing, and that to employ them with children who have useful residual hearing may hinder their use of audition.

Visual Displays

Most visual displays of the speech signal, or certain component parts of it, have been designed as an aid to speech teaching rather than as an aid to speech reception in communication. The exception is the eyeglass display invented by Upton (see bibliography, page 147). The electronic displays most commonly encountered are those which employ an oscilloscope, a television screen, or an array of lights to present patterns that indicate fundamental frequency, duration of voicing, how well the child approximates a vowel target, or how acceptably he produces a certain consonant. Meters are also used to indicate the presence of a fricative such as [s] or a nasal sound such as [m]. More complex arrays that have recently been introduced include one which produces spectrographic patterns as the child talks. These patterns are almost identical to those introduced in Chapter 4.

The function of electronic visual displays is to provide feedback to the child. They can tell him whether his attempt to produce a particular speech pattern has been successful or not. They cannot help the child produce the desired pattern correctly in the first place. For those who need such help, there is no substitute for the skilled teacher/clinician. But the skilled teacher/clinician can also provide visual feedback by simple, non-electronic, means. For example, she can raise or lower her hand to indicate the extent to which the child is modulating the pitch of his voice (F_0). She can move an object on a card, draw a line on a piece of paper, or pull out a carpenter's tape to indicate and measure the duration or intensity of a vocalization. When she hears that he achieves correct production of vowel or consonant target patterns, she can simply reinforce the child by allowing him to amass tokens that can be exchanged for candy. This being so, one must ask what place electronic visual displays might have in a speech teaching program. Because they can provide feedback on speech production in the absence of a teacher/clinician, the most plausible answer appears to be that they could allow the child to practice previously acquired skills independently. If one accepts this answer, then one has to ask the following questions: Does a child need to practice previously acquired speech skills? If so, can a visual display provide adequate feedback for such practice? Are there hazards in providing independent practice through the use of visual feedback devices?

As with all other motor skills, there are four components that are essential for the mastery of speech skills: accuracy, speed, economy of effort, and flexibility of usage. There is certainly need for a child to practice these skills, for once an accurate speech pattern has been evoked and can be repeated reliably, practice is required to develop the remaining components and ensure automaticity of production. Accuracy can be checked and speed of production can certainly be increased through the child's independent use of a visual device if the target is unambiguously specified. Economy of effort may not, however, result from visual feedback. There is nothing in a visual display of the acoustic patterns the child may produce that can indicate to him whether or not he is using abnormal, redundant, muscular effort to achieve his result. Flexibility of usage is also hard to achieve when one uses a visual display. In normal speech communication we say words and sounds differently according to their context. In a variety of situations we give them different stress, duration, intensity, and pitch in order to convey our meaning most efficiently. Practice with a visual display tends to encourage a rigidity rather than a flexibility of performance. In short, of the four components of a motor skill acquisition, visual displays may help only with the first two: accuracy and speed.

Are there hazards of independent practice with visual display? Clearly, yes, if one practices accuracy and speed of production without attention to economy of effort; abnormal mechanisms of production may become habitual, to the detriment of fluency. Consider the following examples. Jaw-assisted production of syllables released with [d] may become automatized when, in fact, the tongue alone should be used. Changes in fundamental voice frequency may not be achieved *independently of vocal intensity* if a simple pitch display is used. An [s], displayed as movement of a needle across a meter, may be produced acceptably in isolation because the child uses greater than normal breath stream to produce the turbulence in order to make the sound. Such an [s] cannot be readily generalized to conversational speech because, in the normal course of production, there is less expenditure of breath. A nasal indicator can be employed to teach the child how to produce [n], but the mere production of [n] may do little to help the child. This is because problems with nasality usually occur, not just as an articulation disorder, but as a symptom of generalized inadequacy of velopharyngeal function. A child may practice a vowel or syllable and be informed by the visual display that his production is correct; yet, unless the display also yields information on laryngeal tone, the child may be learning to produce the pattern with an unacceptable voice. These examples indicate that independent practice of skills can rarely be safely allowed, and that visual displays are probably best considered as aids for use by the skilled teacher/clinician rather than as a means of replacing her. We personally use visual displays only for the purpose of reinforcement and for providing feedback during teaching sessions, but never for unsupervised practice.

Visual Cues

Two types of visual cue systems are commonly used to supplement speechreading: those that provide information which relates directly to the articulation of sound patterns, and those that do not. Systems of the first type are mainly designed to provide prompts on consonant production. For example, the speaker may place his finger on his nose to indicate nasality or move a finger sharply away from the side of the chin to indicate a velar plosive. Since speechreading provides fairly clear information on place of production, such prompts are generally related to manner of production or voicing (see Chapter 4). Systems of the second type employ a number of arbitrarily derived hand configurations and hand positions that, together with speechreading, specify each phoneme. The most frequently used of these systems is Cued Speech. Systems of both types are briefly discussed below.

Visual prompts, because they relate to some aspect of articulation, are useful in teaching a child to produce speech patterns that are partly or wholly inaudible to him. They can also serve to correct a child's pronunciation of an unfamiliar word and be used by a speaker to ensure that the child does not confuse two words that may not be specified by context. For example, "pad" and "bat" look alike on the lips and are equally likely to occur in the context of a ball game in a sentence such as "Do you have a _____ ?" Prompts are, however, too cumbersome to use continuously in connected discourse. Imagine how slowly one would have to speak to a hearing-impaired child, and how badly the rhythm of a sentence would be broken, if prompts were used to specify each consonant in a phrase.

Cued Speech serves to clarify speechreading (reception) rather than speech production. Once it is mastered, it can be used without affecting the rate or rhythm of what is said. Although every phoneme is cued, the hand movements from one sound to the next can be executed smoothly so that they flow together as does coarticulated speech. Experiments have shown that Cued Speech can contribute significantly in speech reception. Words and sentences were both received more accurately when Cued Speech was used with a group of children trained with the system than when they were tested with speechreading alone. These experiments, together with teachers' experience, demonstrate that Cued Speech can substantially assist verbal learning.

Of course, it is unnecessary to use either prompts or cues with children who have sufficient residual hearing to differentiate sounds that look alike on the lips. Whether prolonged and consistent use of prompts and cues could adversely affect such children's ability to develop listening skills is a matter for further research. Although many questions relating to Cued Speech remain to be explored, there is no doubt that it can be used advantageously with totally deaf children and with those who have residual hearing but who cannot, for some reason, use it efficiently.

Touch

We use tactile sensation as a form of feedback when we speak, even though we may not be conscious of doing so. Such sensation is of the utmost importance to those hearing-impaired children to whom certain sounds are inaudible. Whereas the normal-hearing listener develops both auditory and articulatory targets in speech production, the hearing-impaired person can develop only articulatory targets for the sounds he cannot hear. His only guide in the articulation of such sounds is how the movement and contact of the articulators feel. In teaching speech to hearing-impaired children, one must pay close attention to evoking and initially rehearsing sounds in contexts that provide optimally tangible orosensory-motor patterns. Thus [k] is more tangible when produced with a central vowel [ka] than with either the front vowel [ki] or the back vowel [ku].

Touch is not used in speech reception by normal-hearing listeners, but it can be used to advantage in speech reception by hearing-impaired persons. Two forms of tactile cues can be made available to them: those provided by a device that transmits some aspect of speech through skin sensation, and those that involve direct touch.

Devices designed to transmit speech through skin sensation range from a simple, single vibrator to a complex display of several dozen vibrators. Tactile aids that stimulate the skin through small electric currents rather than vibration are also being used experimentally. Up to the present time, the most commonly used tactile device has been a single vibrator driven by a hearing aid. Such a device can increase awareness of sound for a totally deaf child and allow him to use touch as a distance sense. The single vibrator can provide but limited cues, however. It cannot convey the complexities of speech. The skin is relatively insensitive to changes in frequency and to high-frequency sounds. A single vibrator can, therefore, only help a child to discriminate between low-frequency sounds that differ in intensity and duration. Such an aid to discrimination is worthwhile but, since background noise generally has strong low-frequency components, it can be used to advantage only in quiet surroundings.

Research on the tactile transmission of speech is in progress and will hopefully lead to the development of tactile aids that are portable and can supplement speechreading in everyday communication. Their great advantage over visual cues would be two-fold: First, they would reduce the heavy burden already placed on vision by the child's need to speechread and to orient himself to objects and people in his environment; second, because the device would automatically present a representation of the speech pattern to the skin, there would be no need for people to learn a cue system or for the child to function on reduced information when communicating with people who could not provide additional visual cues.

Direct touch can provide a great deal of help to a child in the speech-training session. One can use touch to feel the presence of nasality (vibration of the nose), voice (vibration of the chest), and the turbulence of fricatives (air stream from the mouth). One can also indicate the smoothness of a certain sound by stroking the child's arm, or the sharp release of a plosive by tapping the child's knee. The amount of tension required to produce a certain vowel or consonant can similarly be conveyed by squeezing the child's hand. Thus, touch can help the teacher/clinician to foster speech production through both direct experience and analogy. There are simple ways of using touch in evoking any speech pattern, but tactile prompts should not be used once a speech pattern has been evoked and rehearsed. Like visual prompts, they would impair the speed and rhythm of connected speech. It is not known whether prolonged, regular use of tactile cues and prompts could detract from a child's use of residual audition. It is quite possible that the use of tactile aids could focus the child's attention on touch, rather than hearing. Until this possibility has been explored through research, it would seem wise to us to reserve the use of touch for those children who have little or no useful residual audition. We shall return to our discussion of touch and the other senses in speech acquisition in the next chapter.

ANNOTATED BIBLIOGRAPHY

Berger, K. W.   *Speechreading: Principles and Methods.* Baltimore, Md.: National Educational Press, 1972.
An excellent review of the speechreading process and the studies that have been carried out on visual speech reception, this text is an easy-to-read introduction to the topic.

Fant, G. (Ed.)   *Speech Communication and Profound Deafness.* Washington, D.C.: A. G. Bell Association for the Deaf, 1972.
This book is a collection of papers presented at an international conference of scientists in Sweden in 1970. It includes more extensive discussion of visual cue and visual prompt systems than appears in any other publication. It also contains an abundance of information relevant to many other chapters in the present text.

Jeffers, J., and Barley, M.   *Speechreading.* Springfield, Ill.: Charles C Thomas, 1971.
The principles of speechreading, the visibility (and invisibility) of speech sounds, methods and materials for teaching and testing speechreading are put forward in this well-organized text. The book is intended more as a guide for teachers of adults who lose their hearing than for those working with hearing-impaired children. Accordingly, there is little attention given to the acquisition of verbal skills through vision.

Stark, R. E. (Ed.)   *Sensory Capabilities of Hearing-Impaired Children.* Baltimore, Md.: University Park Press, 1974.
This book is based on the proceedings of a workshop sponsored by the Johns Hopkins University School of Medicine, at which leading

authorities in the field presented papers on various aspects of the senses in speech reception. These papers and the discussion that followed them were included, with the result that this text is the most comprehensive treatment of vision and touch as supplementary or alternative modalities to audition in the acquisition of verbal skills by hearing-impaired children.

Upton, H. W.   Wearable eyeglass speechreading aid. *American Annals of the Deaf,* 113, 222–229, 1968.
 One of a number of articles in this issue of the *American Annals* that describe the range of visual aids available to teachers.

9. Speech: Assessment and Teaching

Speech is man's major means of communication. Inability to speak—or to understand speech—is therefore a serious personal and social handicap. Hearing-impaired children generally have difficulty with some, if not all, aspects of speech acquisition. A child's speech production skills usually reflect the extent to which he is (or has been) deprived of speech training and acoustic information. Thus a totally deaf child will not learn to talk unless he is taught to do so, and a child with residual hearing only in the low-frequency range will not spontaneously master the use of high-frequency speech sounds. Children with hearing levels of 60 to 70 dB over the speech frequencies of 80–8000 Hz cannot hear spoken language at conversational levels and, without hearing aids, will function as if they are totally deaf to speech. Given appropriate hearing aids and sufficient involvement in speech communication, many such children can receive enough acoustic information to acquire speech naturally. The need for speech teaching therefore varies from child to child, principally according to hearing loss. The more severely hearing impaired the child, the more likely it is that he will need to be taught speech production skills.

In a previous publication (D. Ling, 1976), a detailed system for teaching speech production skills to hearing-impaired children was described. In this chapter we shall summarize the main ideas underlying this system, describe the weaknesses, strengths, and difficulties that teacher/clinicians have found in putting it into practice, and indicate how some of the problems associated with the assessment and teaching of speech can be readily overcome.

The goal of teaching speech production skills is to provide the child with the means to express himself fluently and effectively through spoken language in a variety of social situations. Speech teaching is worthless unless it is directed to this goal. Failure to reach this goal is common because speech training is, in general, appallingly inadequate. To be optimally effective, speech training has to begin early, be undertaken frequently and consistently, and be systematically carried out so that it rapidly enables the child to use speech as an efficient means of communication. It must relate closely to his language development. Speech training is facilitated by the utmost use of residual hearing. But even total deafness is not an insuperable barrier to clear speech.

Speech Development

Speech development involves the acquisition of a variety of skills. Analysis of these skills shows that most of them are dependent upon previously acquired behaviors. The most basic skills are those involving respiration and phonation—the ability to control breath and to produce voice at will. Without such basic skills a child cannot produce any vowels reliably. Without the ability to produce a range of vowels, a child cannot produce the variety of consonants that are required for intelligible speech, for few consonants are sounds in their own right. Most, in fact, are simply ways of starting or stopping vowels; the word "consonants" means *with* (con) *vowels* (sonants). Without the ability to produce most simple consonants in syllables, a child cannot produce the consonant blends that many words contain. Thus the word "stop" cannot be said correctly by a child who is unable to produce both an /s/ and a /t/. In short, speech development proceeds sequentially through several broad stages, namely: vocalization, vowels, consonants, and consonant blends, each stage providing a foundation for the next.

As normally hearing children learn to produce sound patterns, they quickly employ them in the act of communication. Thus a baby who can only vocalize will use vocalization to attract attention; an infant who does not have the necessary consonants will produce word approximations using the vowels in his repertoire, and a child who cannot produce consonant blends will use single consonants as substitutes.

Four processes underlie the gradual acquisition of correct speech patterns: cognitive growth, linguistic growth, perceptual development, and increasing motor control (see Chapter 3). A child must have something to say before he can use speech communicatively. He must be able to differentiate sound patterns, and he must be able to control his breath, larynx, jaw, tongue, and lips in order to produce these patterns. Unless a child makes progress in each of these respects, his communicative speech will not improve. This is true of both normally hearing and hearing-impaired children.

Speech training is concerned with the concurrent development of the four processes specified above. None of these four processes should be emphasized at the expense of another. A hearing-impaired child will be forced to use gross approximations to words rather than correct patterns when he speaks if his cognitive and language skills are developed (1) without due attention to the use of his sense modalities—particularly his residual hearing—and/or (2) without regard for his learning motor control in the production of speech patterns. Over time, these approximations will become habitual and hard to modify, for practice does not make perfect—it tends only to make permanent. Similarly, one can impede cognitive and linguistic growth if one concentrates on the perfection of motor patterns—correct production of sounds—without also ensuring that the sounds learned are used in meaningful contexts.

It is rare for normally hearing children to produce speech sounds for the first time in words. Speech sounds are usually produced in vocalization or babble before they occur in communicative speech. Vocalization and babble provide both normally hearing and hearing-impaired children with the opportunity to develop the motor control necessary for speech. At the same time, feedback permits the sound that is vocalized or babbled to be differentiated from other sounds. If a speech pattern only occurs in babble, however, it cannot be considered as acquired. The pattern must be used consistently in the context of meaningful speech before the child can be credited with adequate production skill.

A child passes through at least six steps in learning to produce a given speech pattern. First, he develops the prerequisite behaviors. Second, he learns to produce the sound pattern either in isolation or in a single context. Third, he produces the sound in different contexts, usually during vocal play. Fourth, he tries to use the sound pattern meaningfully in one or two words—not always appropriately. Fifth, he uses the sound pattern correctly in a few words. Finally, he uses the sound pattern correctly and consistently in running speech. Some of these steps may take several weeks or even months, but mastery comes only with practice in situations that provide adequate feedback and reinforcement. At first, the child's conscious effort is required to produce a given sound pattern. As he gains experience with the pattern, his production of it becomes increasingly automatic. Truly fluent speech never requires conscious effort on the part of the speaker.

Normally hearing children do not concentrate on learning the production of one sound pattern at a time. Indeed, it would be uneconomical for them to do so. They play with, and attempt to communicate with, several different patterns during a day or even during one utterance. This allows them to compare old patterns with new and to contrast the various new sounds they are learning to make. When training hearing-impaired children to speak one should follow this same process. If one regards each different sound pattern in speech as a separate target, the production of at least six different targets each day should be encouraged. One target behavior may be the production of a new sound pattern; another may be using a previously evoked sound in a new context; yet another may be the use of familiar targets in words that were formerly accepted as approximations. Nothing could be more boring, and few activities could be so ineffective, as teaching only one or two speech patterns at a time.

Speech Evaluation

Speech evaluation should be undertaken before, during, and after training. Evaluation before training permits one to determine what a child can do and cannot do and thus provides bases for planning an individual's training program. Evaluation during training is needed in order to determine whether the child has learned the skills the teacher/clinician set out to teach or to help the child develop. Evaluation following training is essential to determine whether the child has retained the skills that were taught.

Three forms of evaluation can be used to assess a child's speech production skills: a phonetic level test, a phonologic level test, and an intelligibility test. A phonetic level test is used to determine what sound patterns a child is able to produce at will. This test usually demands the child's imitation of the examiner. A phonologic level test is used to determine what sound patterns the child actually uses in his communicative speech. It thus requires the analysis of a recorded sample of the child's conversation.

Intelligibility tests are used to determine the extent to which the child's speech can be understood by others. Such tests require that a sample of the child's speech be rated by a panel of judges. A child who omits certain sound patterns when speaking spontaneously may do so because he cannot produce these patterns, because he does not know how to pronounce particular words, or because his approximations of given words have been accepted for so long that faulty pronunciation has become habitual. Comparison of phonetic and phonologic level tests allows one to determine whether pronunciation or inability to make the required sound patterns is the root cause of the problem.

Each form of evaluation described above is essential at some point in the course of speech training. Phonetic level testing is appropriate at all times. It allows the teacher/clinician to specify what sound patterns a child can or cannot produce and hence to pinpoint the specific target behaviors that have to be developed. Phonologic level testing is appropriate from the time that the child has begun to use an abundance of utterances to communicate. Carried out every few months, it permits one to determine whether the child spontaneously uses his phonetic level skills in everyday speech, or whether he requires training to do so. Intelligibility tests become appropriate only when the majority of phonetic and phonologic level skills have been mastered.

Phonetic Level Assessment

The design of a phonetic level test poses several problems. In order to test phonetic level skills, all target behaviors at each stage of speech development must be specified. The order in which they are presented in the test must correspond closely with the order in which each should be taught. Given such an arrangement, the first items failed by the child should be among the first to be taught by the teacher/clinician. The phonetic level test presented in *Speech and the Hearing-Impaired Child: Theory and Practice,* pp. 163–169 (D. Ling, 1976), appears to meet this requirement, except in two regards.

First, the test specifies the non-segmental aspects of speech—

control of duration, intensity and pitch—as separate from and preceding differentiated vowel production. Most children do, in fact, learn to control voice patterns before they can produce all vowels. In this respect, the development sequence provided by the evaluation model is acceptable as proposed. However, when older hearing-impaired children who have already acquired some vowels are found to be unable to control voice adequately, the problem is one of remediation rather than one of initial development. In such cases, non-segmental and segmental skills can be evaluated and taught concurrently (D. Ling, 1976, p. 152). In short, when some vowel patterns have already been mastered, it seems preferable to teach control of duration, intensity, and pitch with as many different vowels as possible to develop independent control of the larynx and the articulators in a variety of contexts.

Second, the test specifies vowels as a complete stage preceding the differentiation of consonants. Certainly several vowels must be acquired before consonants can be effectively produced. The question is, "How many?" In the original text (D. Ling, 1976, p. 174), it was suggested that 70 percent of vowels and diphthongs should be taught before work on differentiated consonant production is begun. This proportion appears to be unnecessarily high. The first stage of consonant development can evidently be entered as soon as the child has acquired the vowels and diphthongs specified in the first step, namely [a, i, u, aʊ and aɪ]. Work on the vowels in the second and subsequent steps can then be undertaken, first in the context of consonants differentiated by manner, and then in the context of all other consonants, as originally outlined. Our own work, and that of several teacher/clinicians who have applied the system, indicates that a more rapid shift to consonant production has two advantages: Children can formulate more words correctly at an earlier point in speech acquisition and are thus encouraged to transfer the phonetic skills they have learned into phonological contexts more rapidly; and the short vowels are most easily developed in a consonantal context. Although these points were discussed in the original text (pp. 119, 122 and 239), the test does not reflect such a sequence. It should.

Phonologic Level Assessment

This assessment requires that 50 representative utterances be tape-recorded. On playback, each speech pattern—listed on a printed form—is checked as absent (−), inconsistently present (+), or consistently present (√), (see D. Ling, 1976, pp. 144–147). Two problems related to these procedures have been identified. The first relates to the time-consuming nature of the task; the second concerns the range of inconsistency that may be present as sound patterns are being incorporated into the child's phonology. These problems are discussed below.

Time is taken up in the two steps of the phonologic evaluation: data collection and data analysis. If the child has reached the stage at which a phonologic evaluation is a meaningful measure, the time required for recording 50 representative utterances should not exceed half an hour. If the child speaks or can be stimulated to speak so rarely that fewer than 50 utterances are produced in this time, then emphasis in his program should be upon developing his spoken language and his desire to communicate. To save time in the analysis—the second step of phonologic evaluation—a short form of the evaluation could obviously be administered. Then, instead of listening for the use of all speech patterns on every evaluation, one could listen only for the use of those that the child had acquired at the phonetic level. On initial phonetic level testing, for example, the child might be found to have most vowels and a few consonants. In the short form of the phonologic evaluation, one would determine only whether each of these phonemes was present in his meaningful speech and used with adequate intensity, duration, pitch, and voice quality. On subsequent testing, one would determine whether patterns previously absent or inconsistently used had become a consistent part of his speech, and whether patterns taught since the previous phonetic level test had also become incorporated into his phonology.

The advantage of occasionally using a short form of the phonologic test would be that teacher/clinicians could be expected to undertake evaluation more frequently. Hopefully, more frequent evaluation would tend to focus attention upon the need to ensure that the child transfers whatever patterns he can produce phonetically into his meaningful speech. The extent to which the child uses particular sound patterns in meaningful speech could be indicated on his phonetic level evaluation form. Such a procedure would encourage the teacher/clinician to regard the phonologic use of sound patterns as one or more of the half-dozen targets chosen for the child at any given time.

The use of a short form does not overcome the need for regular, full phonologic evaluation. Children may use a pattern consistently in their phonologic speech at one stage and, later, use it inconsistently or not at all. Such lapses often occur for several reasons: The use of the sound pattern may not have become habitual; a sufficient level of automaticity may not have been reached; the child may not know how to incorporate the sound into new vocabulary; more complex language forms demand greater flexibility in the use of sound patterns. We therefore suggest that a full phonologic evaluation should be undertaken annually, and that a short form of phonologic evaluation be undertaken every two or three months. The teacher/clinician should, at all times, listen for and encourage the phonologic use of the sound patterns she teaches.

To rate a child as making consistent use of a sound pattern in phonologic speech is to state that the child's production of that sound pattern in words and sentences conforms with that of normally speaking children of the same age and background. If the hearing-impaired child's peers normally omit a sound or substitute another in their speech in a fashion typical of normal development or as part of their dialect, then the hearing-impaired child should be regarded as having consistent use of a sound pattern if he does the same. One can only regard anything less than 100 percent normal usage of a sound pattern as unacceptable. Assume, for example, that one accepted a criterion of 80 percent correct production in a sample of phonologic speech. This would mean that one regarded 20 percent error as acceptable. If every phoneme used was wrongly produced or omitted 20 percent of the time, then a child's speech would be unintelligible. To specify 100 percent normal production as one's criterion for consistent phonologic use nevertheless leads to the rating of any sound pattern as "inconsistent" if it is used correctly between one and 99 percent of the time. Is such a rating too broad to be useful? We think not, because inconsistent usage demands that the teacher/clinician pay attention to the child's production of that pattern.

Of course, there are levels of inconsistency. A child who makes correct use of a sound pattern 80 percent of the time is more advanced than the child who uses it correctly only 20 percent of the time. It is possible to measure the extent of inconsistency with frequently occurring sound patterns, such as most vowels and simple consonants, and hence to chart progress toward their consistent use. However, some sound patterns, such as certain consonant blends, are unlikely to occur more than once or twice, if at all, in a phonologic sample of 50 representative utterances. To rate levels of inconsistency of usage cannot, therefore, be meaningful except in the early stages of speech development. Certainly, the teacher/clinician who can afford the time should analyze and calculate the proportion of times a phoneme is used correctly relative to omissions, distortions, and substitutions. Such a procedure may, however, have more value in research than in teaching.

Intelligibility Tests

To test the intelligibility of a child's speech before he is able to consistently produce most sound patterns is as futile as asking a child to sprint when he can barely walk. Intelligibility tests are much more time-consuming than any other measure of speech because they require the participation of a panel of judges as well as that of the child and teacher/clinician. The most popular form of intelligibility test is that in which the child reads the test material. Such a test is not so much one of meaningful speech, but one of oral reading skills. The outcome of such tests largely depends on how the child has been taught and whether or not the judges are familiar with the speech of hearing-impaired children. Intelligibility tests may, in carefully controlled research studies, yield useful comparative data. However, one can rarely predict on the basis of such tests how well a child will be understood by the strangers he is likely to meet in everyday life.

Once a child has a reasonable command of language and his phonetic and phonologic skills enable him to produce most speech patterns (including some consonant blends), it becomes possible to measure the intelligibility of his spontaneous speech. Such a measure can provide unique information. It can indicate how well words are blended and sentences are phrased, whether words in sentences are produced to accord with the stress-timed patterns of English, and whether intonation and stress are used to provide semantic cues. In short, tests of the intelligibility of spontaneous speech, judged by skilled teacher/clinicians, can show whether the child can adequately integrate the suprasegmental and segmental aspects of production. Phonetic and phonologic level tests cannot provide this information. Intelligibility tests based on spontaneous speech and judged by listeners who are unfamiliar with hearing-impaired children are, of course, the most rigorous measure of a child's speaking skills.

Speech and Residual Audition

The most efficient way to develop speech is through the use of residual hearing. Conversely, one of the most efficient ways to develop auditory discrimination skills is through the teaching of speech. Given appropriate hearing aids, most hearing-impaired children will be able to hear, and learn to control the most fundamental aspect of speech production—the presence or absence of vocalization. How much more of speech a child will be able to hear and learn to produce will depend mainly upon the extent of residual hearing. The majority of children whose hearing levels over the frequencies 125 to 4000 Hz are 70 dB or better, can be expected to acquire most, if not all, speech patterns without specific teaching—*if* they are provided with appropriate hearing aids and given sufficient auditory experience. The extent to which hearing levels are more severe than about 70 dB and the extent to which frequency range of hearing is limited toward the low-frequency end of the speech spectrum (to the left of the audiogram), largely determine how likely it is that speech teaching and speech discrimination training will be required by a child.

Speech is a concrete event. When a child vocalizes, says a word, or produces a sentence, there is no doubt that he has done so on the part of the listener. Hearing, on the other hand, is not an overt, concrete behavior. One may speak without the child giving any indication of having heard or understood. Thus speech development is easier to promote and to track than auditory development. One can reinforce a speech event immediately. But one can only reinforce the child for having detected, discriminated, identified, or understood something through hearing if or when he responds in some way. Because a child's spontaneous acquisition of a speech pattern and his direct imitation of a sound are clear evidence that accurate auditory discriminations have been made, both are good measures of the use of residual hearing. Both also provide opportunity to reinforce the child's use of audition. Although spontaneous speech acquisition and imitation provide good evidence of auditory discrimination skill, there is usually a significant lag between auditory discrimination and speech production in the early stages of development. Auditory skills and speech skills do not develop in parallel. Normal-hearing infants can discriminate between sounds that they cannot initially produce, and the same is true for many hearing-impaired children. The lag is greater between discrimination and production of consonants than between discrimination and production of voice patterns, i.e., suprasegmental features.

Discrimination is but a special case of detection. In measuring detection, one is concerned with the child's ability to hear whether a sound is present. With discrimination, one is concerned with the child's ability to detect a difference between sounds. Such abilities are necessary, but not sufficient, for the spontaneous development or imitation of speech. The child must additionally develop the motor skills to produce a sound pattern and the auditory memory span that will permit him to compare his own production with that of others.

In an auditory approach to speech teaching, one must allow for the fact that auditory processing of speech is not an overt, concrete behavior, and that speech production will normally lag behind speech discrimination skills. One must be prepared to provide the child with abundant auditory experience before expecting the development or imitation of particular speech patterns. One can, however, minimize the lag by ensuring that the child's vocalizations and speech (and hence his acquisition of motor control over the mechanisms of production) are encouraged. The more reinforcement a child receives, the more frequently and extensively he will use voice and speech.

The process of speech acquisition is one of progressive differentiation and control of motor movements and increasing conformity with the phonology of the community. *If the hearing-impaired child is using his residual audition in the acquisition of speech, there should be a continuous, perceptible growth in the quantity and variety of sound patterns that he produces from one week to the next.* Guided by hearing, vocalization should become more varied in intensity, duration, and pitch as the child experiments with his voice. Distinct vowels should emerge from vocalization and gradually increase in variety to include those produced high in the front [i] and high at the back [u] of the mouth (see Chapter 4). Consonants should begin to be used as vowels are acquired, first randomly and then systematically as tongue control is developed. Failure to progress within a particular stage of development or to progress from one stage to the next, indicates either that the child's hearing aid is inappropriate, that he is not receiving adequate auditory stimulation and reinforcement, that he is reaching the limits imposed by his residual hearing, or that there are problems in addition to hearing impairment that prevent or hinder speech development. Careful evaluation is required to pinpoint the cause.

Audition and Voice Patterns

The speech patterns that a child can first produce, which are varied vocalizations, involve relatively gross motor control. Although acoustic cues on duration, intensity, and pitch occur throughout the whole frequency range of speech, residual hearing for low frequencies is sufficient for their discrimination. This is indicated by reference to Figure 9.1, which is a narrow-band spectrogram of the word "hello" spoken by a female adult, first in a monotone and then with marked intonation. If one places a paper horizontally across the spectrogram so that only those patterns that lie below 1000 Hz are visible, one can see that they have different properties. The first is shorter than the second, indicat-

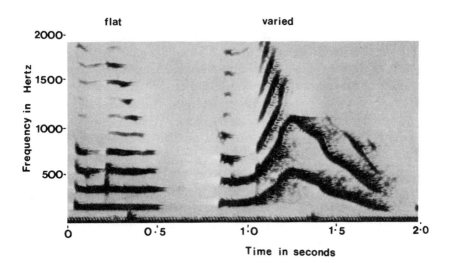

Figure 9.1

A narrow-band spectrogram of the word hello *spoken by a female adult using flat and varied intonation patterns. The acoustic energy reflecting change in voice pitch is shown to be distributed over a wide range of frequencies.*

ing that differences in duration should be audible to children with hearing only below this frequency. The second is also darker than the first, indicating that its intensity was greater. In the first, the harmonics (see Chapter 4) are seen as straight, horizontal bars; this indicates that the word was spoken in a monotone. In the second, the harmonics are seen to rise and fall in frequency, which indicates how intonation was used. If one similarly places a paper horizontally across the spectrogram so that only those patterns below 500 Hz are visible, distinct differences between the two pronunciations of the world "hello" can still be seen.

That differences between speech patterns can be seen on a spectrogram does not guarantee that they will be audible to a hearing-impaired child. In order for such a child to hear these differences, the hearing aid must amplify sounds over the frequency range in which the patterns occur, and the child must have the capacity to differentiate them. The capacity to differentiate and to reproduce voice patterns that vary in intensity and duration can be expected of most children, even those whose responses to low-frequency sounds are tactile rather than auditory in origin. The capacity to differentiate patterns that vary in frequency is, in general, related to the amount of residual hearing present under 1000 Hz. Most children with hearing up to and beyond 1000 Hz can be expected to have, or to develop, sufficiently fine pitch discrimination to hear and produce small variations in voice pitch—and even to sing in tune—if they have appropriate hearing aids. The minimal requirement is that one or two harmonics of the vocal pattern are audible. Children whose hearing is more restricted may not be able to discriminate fine variations in voice pitch. For example, those whose hearing extends up to about 500 Hz and those who respond only when sound produces a tactile (vibratory) sensation may only perceive differences in pitch of voice when they vary by half an octave or more.

Children who are hearing-impaired usually produce varied voice patterns during their first year of life. If they have useful residual hearing and are fitted with appropriate hearing aids at this stage, natural voice quality and variation of voice patterns can usually be preserved without specific auditory or speech training. The later the child with severe or profound hearing impairment receives a hearing aid, the more likely it is that his range of vocalization will be restricted and that he will require specific training in the discrimination and production of voice patterns. The two as-

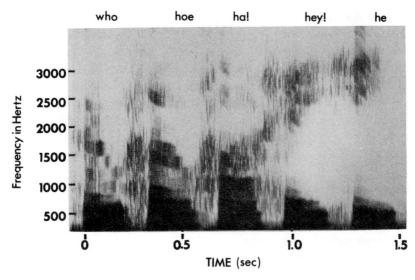

who   hoe   ha!   hey!   he

Figure 9.2
A broad-band spectrogram of the words who, hoe, ha!, hey!, *and* he *spoken by an adult female, showing how the frequency of the second formants differentiates one from another.*

pects of training—discrimination and production—should be undertaken concurrently. At the outset, grossly different vocalizations should be presented and their production reinforced. Just as many mothers of normal-hearing babies employ exaggerated patterns of intonation in speaking to them, so should teacher/clinicians and parents use a wide range of pitch when they begin to train a hearing-impaired child. Singing to the child and encouraging the child to sing are appropriate at all stages, but particularly so at the beginning of training. As the child responds differentially to, and begins to produce, widely divergent patterns, so can the magnitude of patterns used be gradually reduced. Such training must, of course, be provided as an adjunct to auditory-verbal experience. The child must also use an appropriate hearing aid, be exposed to abundant spoken language, and be encouraged to use voice and speech at all times.

Children who cannot spontaneously learn, or be trained, to control their voice patterns through the use of residual hearing, can be trained to produce sounds varying in intensity, duration, and pitch through the use of visual aids or through touch. We shall discuss such training later on in this chapter.

Audition and Vowels

In order to identify all vowels through audition, a child's residual hearing must extend up to about 2500 Hz, the approximate center frequency of F_2 of the vowel [i] (see Chapter 4). All vowels can be heard if hearing extends up to 1000 Hz or so, but some may sound rather alike because some front and back vowels have similiar F_1 values. These points are illustrated in Figure 9.2, which is a broad-band spectrogram showing five of the English vowels, / u, o, a, e and i /, as they are spoken by a female, in the words *who, hoe, ha!, hey!,* and *he.* The remaining vowels occupy intermediate positions over the frequency range. The nature of the information available below any given frequency may be determined by placing a paper horizontally across the spectrogram and comparing one vowel with another.

All vowels and diphthongs are usually differentiated and produced spontaneously by children whose residual hearing extends up to or beyond 2500 Hz, providing that appropriate hearing aids are worn from early in life, and that ample auditory-verbal experience is provided. Children with no hearing above 500 Hz cannot be expected to differentiate more than one or two vowels through audition alone. Those with hearing up to about 1000 Hz can usually discriminate only between vowels that have dissimilar first formants if they are presented in isolation. However, when vowels with similar first formants are released with consonants such as [b, w and m] that are audible to the child with hearing up to 1000 Hz, consonant-to-vowel transitions may provide sufficient cues for the auditory discrimination and identification of all vowels. Differences in the /h/ preceding the vowels depicted in Figure 9.2 provide an example of the additional information available for their identification when they are produced in the context of certain consonants.

Specific training in the auditory recognition and production of vowels is likely to be required by children whose residual hearing does not extend up to about 2500 Hz. The more restricted the frequency range of audition, the more likely it is that the child will need to use vision as a supplement or as an alternative to audition. Whereas speechreading provides no direct information on voice patterns, it can help a child to discriminate between vowels in speech reception. Speechreading is, however, a poor guide to the child in speech production. It provides clear information on jaw and lip positions, but little or no indication of tongue placement, which is crucial in producing the formant structure of vowels. Since residual audition extending up to 1000 Hz can provide information on the location of all first formants, the acquisition of vowels is best fostered in children with low-frequency residual audition by ensuring that their attention is not focused exclusively upon speechreading, but that sufficient attention is paid to audible components. Failure in this regard leads to the production of a neutral vowel regardless of lip and jaw position. Such neutralization, a common fault among hearing-impaired children, is frequently met with the vowel [i]. If attention is directed to the audible as well as the visible components of this vowel, then the presence of a high, rather than a low, first formant should be audible to a child with residual hearing up to 1000 Hz when the vowel is neutralized.

Teaching a child with low-frequency residual hearing to discriminate and produce all vowels is much easier when the child has first learned to discriminate voice pitch. This is because pitch discrimination is an essential element in the differentiation of vowels. Indeed, if a child neutralizes vowels, it is often useful to begin a training session on vowel production with a brief spell of pitch discrimination and pitch production in order to focus the child's attention upon the use of his residual hearing.

Auditory discrimination of vowels normally precedes their production. In most cases, the child's awareness of acoustic differences between his own production and that of others will encourage the child to experiment with and produce an increasingly wide range of vowels. To expect this sequence of events among older children with a very restricted range of residual hearing is not always realistic. In some such cases, auditory discrimination of vowels may best be fostered by first teaching the child to produce the various vowel sounds, perhaps by tactile strategies. Thus armed with the awareness that differences among vowels do exist, such children may more readily search for the acoustic cues by which vowels in their repertoire may be differentiated.

Audition and Consonants

Acoustic cues on manner of consonant production occur throughout the frequency range of speech. However, sufficient cues for the identification of semi-vowels, nasals, and plosives are present even below 500 Hz. This fact is illustrated in Figure 9.3, which is a spectrogram showing the three syllables [wa], [ma], and

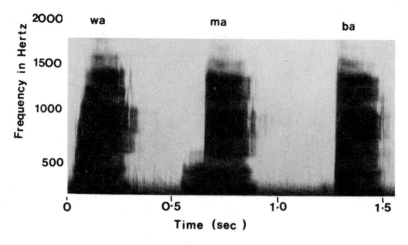

Figure 9.3

A broad-band spectrogram of the syllables [wa], [ma], *and* [ba], *spoken by an adult female, illustrating the marked differences in onset and consonant-to-vowel transitions that differentiate between them. The differences under 500 Hz that can be seen on the spectrogram can usually be heard even by children with only low-frequency residual audition.*

[ba]. In the first syllable, the slope to the left of the spectrogram indicates the low-frequency glide that uniquely specifies a semi-vowel. In the second syllable, the strong formant below 300 Hz preceding the vowel, and the distinct onset of the vowel itself, uniquely specify a nasal consonant. The sharp onset of the third syllable, a perpendicular line on the spectrogram, clearly specifies a voiced plosive. Of course, certain manners of consonant production cannot be identified unless residual hearing extends well beyond 1000 Hz. Thus, unvoiced fricatives other than [h] contain no low-frequency energy, and affricates such as [tʃ] contain only weak components under 1000 Hz.

Manner distinctions among consonants classed as semi-vowels, nasals, or plosives are signaled as much by their onset characteristics, which vary in time, as by their formant frequencies (see Figure 9.3). For this reason, they are relatively easy for most children—even those with limited low-frequency hearing—to discriminate. In training children to produce such distinctions, therefore, it is rarely necessary to employ a sense other than hearing. Indeed, the nasals and the plosives cannot be reliably differentiated through vision. The common confusion of [b] and [m]

in the speech of hearing-impaired children, as in the neutralization of vowels, usually reflects inadequate use of residual audition
and undue emphasis on the child's use of vision. In short, such
confusion is more likely to be due to inappropriate teaching strategies of the teacher/clinician than to the child's actual capacity to
differentiate these sounds through hearing.

Teaching a child to discriminate and produce manner distinctions should be complementary procedures. Production serves to
foster discrimination of the acoustic cues that differentiate one
manner of production from another, and vice versa. Optimum
discrimination and production of these consonant distinctions are
promoted by teaching them in units of at least syllabic length.
Only in the context of a vowel can the essential differences between one sound and another become fully apparent. Thus, if the
[m] is taught in isolation, the child will not learn to recognize the
sudden and distinctive formant shift that occurs at the onset of the
vowel (see Figure 9.3). Since this rapid formant shift will not occur
if the child nasalizes the vowel, his auditory recognition of the
distinction and his ability to produce it are of considerable importance in his acquisition of velopharyngeal control (see D. Ling,
1976, pp. 248–252).

Unlike manner distinctions, place of consonant production
cannot be discriminated by children who have only low-frequency
residual hearing. Most acoustic cues on place of production lie
between 1500 and 3000 Hz. Thus, unless children have residual
hearing for these frequencies they will be unable to differentiate
consonants that vary in their place of production. The consonants [b], [d], and [g] will tend to sound alike to the child who
has residual hearing only below 1000 Hz, as will [m], [n] and [ŋ],
or [p], [t] and [k]; no amount of auditory training will make them
sound significantly different to such children. Of course, those
with residual hearing up to 3000 Hz may require specific training
in the reception and production of the high-frequency sounds. If
so, such training should always be provided in the context of
syllables or words so that both variant and invariant acoustic cues
on place of production come to be recognized. Children without
such hearing invariably have to be taught how to produce high-
frequency sounds through the simultaneous use of more than one
sense modality. Hearing alone is inadequate in such cases.

The scanty nature of the place cues that lie below 1500 Hz is
shown in the spectrogram of the three syllables [pa], [ta], and [ka]

presented as Figure 9.4. There are slight differences in voice onset time (the lag between release of the plosion and the onset of voicing) in these syllables, as evidenced by the space between the perpendicular line (the plosive) and the mass of energy (the vowel). However, these differences are not usually sufficiently distinctive for place discrimination among consonants.

Voice onset time is a crucial variable in differentiating voiced from unvoiced plosives such as [b] and [p]. In voiced sounds, the vocal cords vibrate at about the same time as the plosive is released (see [ba] in Figure 9.3), whereas there is a substantial lag between plosion and voicing in unvoiced consonants (see [pa] in Figure 9.4). In order to teach children to discriminate and produce the voiced/voiceless distinction in consonants, it is often useful initially to exaggerate and then to reduce the voice onset time of unvoiced plosives and the duration of unvoiced fricatives so that the child readily perceives the nature of the distinction. Such a prop should not, of course, be allowed to become habitual. To prevent abnormal prolongation of voicelessness if such a strategy has to be used,

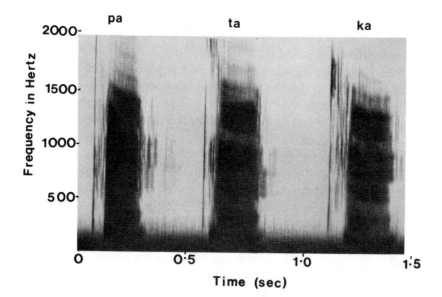

Figure 9.4
A broad-band spectrogram of the syllables [pa], [ta], *and* [ka], *spoken by an adult female, showing that there is very little information below 1500 Hz for their auditory discrimination if only low-frequency residual hearing is present.*

the child should be required to discriminate and produce several syllables repeated rapidly — for example, [pa, pa, pa] versus [ba, ba, ba] rather than [pa] versus [ba]. The voiced/voiceless distinction can usually be heard and made by children with only low-frequency residual hearing if they are taught to produce unvoiced plosives and unvoiced fricatives before their voiced cognates.

Speech Teaching

Children produce vocalizations spontaneously during their first year of life regardless of the degree of their hearing impairment. Those who have hearing aids at this stage of development can usually be expected to preserve the natural quality and extend the variety of their vocalizations providing that they are encouraged to do so and that they are exposed to an abundance of spoken language. Even totally deaf children can be made aware of their vocalizations through the use of a hearing aid, as vibrations are produced by the hearing aid receiver at high intensity levels. In early treatment the task is to preserve the quality of vocalization present and to extend its variety. In short, early intervention can eliminate the need to teach voice production.

The quantity and quality of spontaneous vocalization produced by a child who cannot hear his own and others' speech tends to decrease rapidly from about 6 months of age. By his second birthday, such a child may have become silent except for the involuntary voicing that occurs in such behaviors as laughing or crying. The use of hearing aids may be sufficient to restore the use of spontaneous vocalization. In the event that it is not, specific training is required to teach the child how to vocalize at will.

One can usually initiate voluntary production of vocalization by exciting the child and reinforcing the involuntary vocalizations that he then produces. Vocalizations occur most readily (and hence opportunities to reinforce them are most frequent) in active play. Various types of reinforcement can be effective. Imitation of, and showing pleasure at, the sounds the child makes, and moving a toy toward the child when a sound is produced, are among the many activities that are effective with young children. With older children, much more varied types of reinforcement can be used. Older children like to have the duration and pitch of their vocalizations measured by seeing how much string can be gradually pulled out of a box, or how far a carpenter's tape can be extended as they vocalize; or how long, how high, or how low a line representing their vocalization can be drawn on a chalkboard before they run out of breath. They also like to see how loud the teacher/clinician or parent requires their vocalization to be before they will release a jack-in-the-box or wake up from a feigned sleep. The range and number of simple reinforcing activities that can be used depend only upon the ingenuity of the adults involved and the materials that are at hand.

Teaching specific speech patterns should not be attempted before abundant vocalization has been established, because production of speech depends upon the presence of adequate breath and voice and the child's ability to control them. Once the child is able to vocalize with ease and uses vocalization as a rudimentary means of communication—whether he has acquired these abilities spontaneously or through training—one should seek to extend the variety of vowel sounds he produces. As soon as a variety of vowels can be produced with natural voice quality, consonants can be introduced in the order indicated earlier. At no time should breath and voice control be ignored. Thus, while teaching vowels or consonants, an adequate reservoir of breath and a good quality voice must be insisted upon. We have previously recommended that a child should be able to produce consonants in syllables at the rate of at least three per second—but of course he must be able to produce more than three syllables on one breath. Without adequate oral breath flow, the orosensory-motor patterns associated with the various speech sounds will be weak and therefore harder for the child to differentiate and to learn.

It is always best to extend a child's range of speech patterns informally through play, since pleasant voice quality tends to predominate in informal situations. New voice patterns can often be evoked in play simply by encouraging the child to produce an abundance of vocalization and reinforcing the desired pattern when it appears. For example, when vocalizing abundantly in certain play situations, a child tends to produce high- and low-pitched voice quite spontaneously. Drawing the child's attention to his variations in voice pitch and having him repeat them is the

Figure 9.5 (opposite): *An analysis of the ways in which the various sense modalities can be employed in teaching particular speech patterns (see text for discussion).*

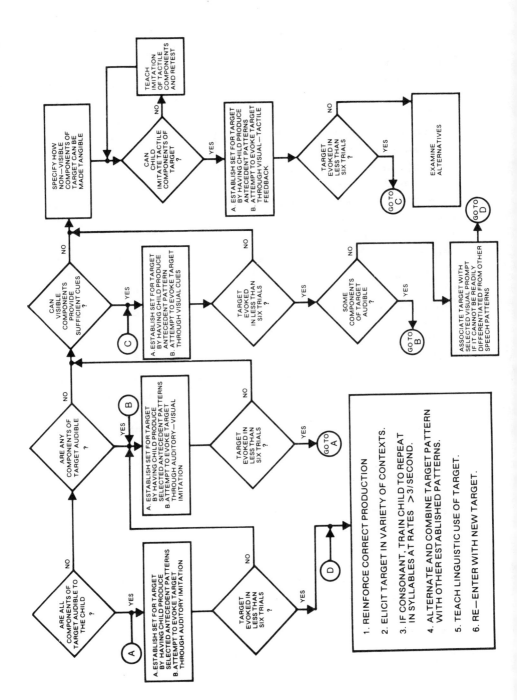

most effective way to establish voice pitch control. Similarly, when promoting abundant vocalization in play, the child will tend to increase the range of vowels and consonants he uses, particularly if the teacher/clinician or parent provides distinct models. Reinforcement and repetition of a new vowel or consonant when the child produces it "by accident" will tend to promote its use on subsequent occasions. An informal approach to speech development should not be an unsystematic approach. Even in an informal approach, the child should be encouraged to produce sound patterns for which the antecedent behaviors have been established—those that have been selected as target patterns on the basis of phonetic and phonologic assessment (see above). Formal teaching is required with children from about 3 years of age when an informal approach fails to yield the production of a speech subskill in a matter of days. We specify days rather than weeks because, at all stages, one is seeking very small, clearly defined, increments in skill.

The sense one must use in order to encourage the development of new voice patterns, vowels, or consonants will, of course, vary from child to child, principally according to the extent of their residual hearing. The task analysis depicted as Figure 9.5 indicates how one can decide upon the strategies that are most appropriate for any given individual. Although this task analysis was designed as a guide in formal teaching, the principles underlying the choice of sense modality also are applicable in informal speech development. In following this task analysis, the reader will find the key questions—which must be answered "Yes" or "No"—in the diamond-shaped cells. Responses to these questions lead, as the arrows indicate, to a further question or instructions contained in rectangles.

The first step in formulating a strategy for teaching a selected target behavior—a subskill of speech—is to determine whether all essential components of the sound pattern selected are audible to the child. If they are, then the answer to the first question in Figure 9.5 is "Yes," and an auditory strategy should be employed (see instructions in the rectangle below the first question). If the target behavior is evoked in less than six trials, then it should be reinforced, elicited in a variety of contexts, etc., as described in the rectangle at the bottom left of this Figure. If it is not evoked in less than six trials, then an auditory-visual strategy should be adopted.

An auditory-visual strategy should be directly adopted in teaching any speech pattern in which one or more of the essential components are inaudible to a child. Thus, an essential component of the [i] vowel, the second formant, would be inaudible to a child with no hearing beyond 1000 Hz. Following the procedure specified in Figure 9.5, when teaching [i] to such a child one would answer the first question 'No" and, following the arrow to the right, answer the second question "Yes." If [i] were evoked through an auditory-visual strategy, one would then proceed to evoke the sound through audition alone. If it were not thus evoked, one would teach it through a tactile-visual strategy, then evoke it through the use of vision alone, vision plus audition, and finally, if the child has hearing for the first formant, through audition alone.

Visual cues alone are usually inadequate for teaching a new sound pattern, as the crucial articulatory features of most speech patterns are invisible. Although lip and jaw positions for a vowel may be visible, tongue position is masked by lips and teeth except in exaggerated models. After a given vowel is learned, normal lip and jaw positions can provide sufficient cues for its imitation, since lip and jaw positions are closely associated with tongue position in English. Further, lip and jaw positions, together with audition of the first formant, uniquely specify a vowel. Visual feedback can, of course, be completely neglected in speech teaching, as evidenced by the acquisition of speech by deaf-blind children who are taught by the Tadoma (touch) method. We do not, obviously, propose that vision should be excluded, but use this example to emphasize that its role must be supportive rather than primary in speech production. The orosensory-motor patterns that are created as the child correctly produces sound patterns are the child's most reliable guide to speech production.

The strategy to be adopted in order to teach sounds that a child cannot hear at all is also indicated in Figure 9.5. Let us assume that a child has no residual hearing above 1000 Hz and that [f] is to be developed. In this case, the answer to the first two questions would certainly be "No." We should also have to answer the third question in the same way because, although the positions of the lips and teeth are visible in [f], the turbulence of the breath stream is not. It is, however, tangible. Thus the child can be expected to place his teeth and lips correctly through vision and to feel the required breath stream on his finger. (There is a simple tactile strategy for teaching every sound pattern of English.) Once the sound has been evoked and the need to produce a turbulent breath stream has been established by means of repetition, there should be no further difficulty in developing [f] through the stages specified in the rectangle at Figure 9.5's lower left corner.

The orosensory-motor patterns associated with [f] are quite unlike those of any other speech sound. The child who has developed these patterns can therefore differentiate [f] from all other sounds that he produces, even though he cannot hear the sound. If the child has hearing up to 1000 Hz, he can differentiate the [f] and the [v] in speech production not only on the basis of orosensory-motor information but also through audition. He can discern the voicing in the [v] and the lack of voicing in the [f] through his residual hearing. In speech production and in speech reception he therefore has an advantage over a totally deaf child. The advantage is greatest in speech reception, since the visible components of [f] and [v] are identical. The same holds true for all voiced/voiceless pairs of consonants.

In everyday speech, context provides many cues that allow the speechreader to differentiate visually similar pairs (see Chapter 8). However, there are many occasions in speech reception when a totally deaf child has no means of knowing whether one or another consonant should be used. It is, therefore, helpful if totally deaf children are provided with visual prompts that unambiguously specify sounds that are visually similar (see rectangle at low-center of Figure 9.5). Prompts that lead to unambiguous speech reception can be provided in many ways. They can relate to some aspect of articulation, such as placing a finger on the nose to differentiate [n] from [d], or touching the chest to indicate voicing, or they can be part of a more formal, abstract system such as Cued Speech (see Chapter 8). We do not advise the use of prompts or cues with children who can function without them.

The most intriguing rectangle in Figure 9.5 is the one at the bottom right of the diagram. This task analysis was designed for teacher/clinicians like ourselves who frequently have to (and often prefer to) work without technological devices other than hearing aids. Alternative strategies therefore abound. There are various visual speech teaching aids, such as nasality indicators, [s] indicators, pitch indicators, and formant frequency displays. Tactile aids are also being created. The potential of such devices has yet to be determined. It is, however, a rare child who, given excellent teaching, fails to produce a speech target for which the prerequisite antecedent behaviors have been adequately established. Among the children from whom a range of target patterns cannot be readily evoked are those with multiple handicaps such as dysarthria, dyspraxia, and severe mental retardation. Specific problems with plosives and fricatives are likely to be experienced by children who have cleft palates; those who have lost their front teeth might have temporary trouble with sibilants and affricates.

In the presence of severe and permanent additional disorders, one may decide that effective speech skills cannot be taught and that alternative means of communication should be fostered. In other cases, one may decide to teach alternative target patterns and to accept that a particular range of speech sounds will be missing from the child's phonology. In yet other instances, one might temporarily neglect a sound pattern—for example, leave an [ʃ] or an [s] until the child's permanent front teeth have grown. Causes of failure, however, often lie with the teacher/clinician rather than with the child. The alternatives in such a case would be to improve the teacher/clinician's competencies or to have a more highly skilled person work with the child.

Conservation and Normalization of Speech

Many children who have the phonetic level skills required to produce highly intelligible speech fail to transfer these skills into their spontaneous expression. There are several possible reasons for such failure: Expectation levels of the teacher/clinician and/or parents may be too low; the child may have inadequate language skills; or the child may not have learned the rules governing the timing of speech patterns in phonologic contexts. Even among children who once had acquired highly intelligible—perhaps normal—speech, standards of production may decline to the point at which it is difficult to understand what they are trying to say. Such may be the case with a child who becomes hearing-impaired after having learned to speak. These problems are discussed below.

Conservation of Speech
Two major modes of feedback are available to the normal-hearing speaker: hearing and orosensory-motor sensation. Fur-

thermore, when speech has been acquired, it is governed as much by feedforward as by feedback mechanisms (see Chapter 8). Thus, when a person loses hearing after having learned spoken language, he should not also lose the ability to speak. Speech can be maintained in a child who loses all hearing—say as the result of meningitis—providing that he is made aware that the feedforward processes he has acquired still work for him and that feedback is still available to him through reference to the oro-sensory-motor patterns created as he speaks. Such awareness requires (1) that the child be encouraged to talk as much as, or even more often than he did before he lost his hearing, and (2) that he is made to realize that his speech, though it may sound different to him, is still intelligible to others.

Sudden loss of hearing, whether partial or total, is a devastating experience for a child. How he speaks is initially less important than how he feels, and how he can learn to understand the speech of others. If he is completely deprived of audition, he can scan the environment only with vision. He can no longer be aware of impending danger through audition. Dozens of things in his daily life lead to an overwhelming sense of insecurity. Only when he has regained a sense of security, and confidence in himself and in others is restored, can speech conservation become a meaningful activity for him.

Fortunately, total loss of hearing due to sickness or accidents is relatively rare. In most cases some residue of hearing remains. If the child has any residual hearing, immediate attention should be given to the selection and fitting of hearing aids, for their use may considerably reduce the severity of the child's problems with speech and adjustment to his handicap. Auditory training and auditory experience are basic requirements, since if the child can hear speech and environmental sounds, at all, they will have a different quality than formerly. He will need to learn how to interpret sound patterns anew. Learning to hear how he speaks should be part of his auditory training.

The child who loses all hearing should receive help from a skilled teacher/clinician immediately. Her first concern should be with the child's adjustment and the part that promoting his understanding of speech can play in fostering adjustment. While learning to speechread is essentially part of the language learning process among children born with hearing impairment, learning such a skill must be regarded as an activity in its own right for children who become totally deaf. Teaching such children to speechread should be based on the principles described in Chapter 8. Usually, if language has already been acquired, speechreading skill can be developed to high levels of efficiency in a relatively short time. Continuation in regular home and school life with additional tutoring is a realistic goal for the majority of children who lose hearing through illness or accident after they have acquired language.

Normalization of Speech

A child's achievements are pervasively influenced by what adults expect of him and how they react to what he does. Only if the adults in a child's family, social, and educational environments expect him to speak intelligibly—a reasonable expectation for most hearing-impaired children—will he ever learn to do so. What is expected of a child must be realistically related to his sensory, intellectual, and social development. Thus expectations for a child must change as the child matures and as he learns. What is acceptable in a child's performance and an adult's response at one stage may not be so at another. In many instances, the greatest obstacle to the normalization of a child's speech is not his capacity to learn, but the difficulty experienced by his teacher/clinician and by his parents in modifying their expectations to accord with his changing abilities.

In the early stages of speech development the adults must learn how to interpret a child's grossly inaccurate approximations to sounds, words, and sentences if the child is to be encouraged to talk at all. To do this, they must be prepared to search for every cue provided by situation and context in order to understand the child, just as he has to use such cues to understand others. That the child can successfully make himself understood with his inadequate repertoire of sounds from the outset is crucially important both to his emotional adjustment and to the development of further speech skills. A child cannot, however, be permitted to rely upon sympathetic adults (or kind-hearted peers) to interpret his impoverished speech when he is capable of producing more richly varied and accurate patterns. Gradually, as the child learns speech skills, so must responsibility for his using them and being understood shift from the caring adult to the child himself. Unless responsibility for his speech (as for other aspects of behavior) is assumed by the child, his progress toward verbal independence will be unnecessarily restricted.

To ensure that the child does eventually assume full responsibility for the quality and intelligibility of his speech, the adult must be ready to say to the child who is capable of a better performance, "I'm sorry, I didn't understand that." Such a strategy is more likely to yield better speech and less hard feeling than direct criticism couched in terms such as, "I know you can do better than that. Say it again" or "You aren't saying your [s] and you're speaking too quietly." After all, an apology and an admission of failure to understand are usually quite acceptable because they imply a possibility of fault in the listener and a concern with the speaker and what he has said. Of course, too frequent and too early use of such a strategy can, like direct criticism, discourage a child to the point of silence. However, its judicious use can be very effective, for to be understood on first hearing when one has something to say provides one with considerable incentive to use clear speech.

There is a risk that children of school age will more often fail to transfer phonetic level skills into phonologic speech when they are taught speech by a specialist than when they are taught speech by their teachers. If taught by a specialist, the child may tend to regard speech as separate from, rather than an integral part of, his everyday school life. Second, the teacher may feel that the child's speech is not her responsibility. Third, the teacher may not be sufficiently aware of what speech skills the child has learned and hence cannot insist upon their use in class. Even when teachers carry out their own speech evaluations and teaching, they may tend to divorce speech from other activities and hence miss many opportunities to insist on correct production of speech patterns in the course of other lessons. The older the child and the longer he has used approximations to words, the more necessary it becomes for the teacher to insist upon the correct use of newly acquired patterns in everyday speech. Failure to insist upon correct use of speech skills in all activities is tantamount to teaching the child that speech lessons and speech itself are irrelevant to everyday life. Hearing-impaired children who attend special schools do so because they have a communication problem. It follows that the amelioration of each aspect of this problem must be given high priority in all facets of their education.

A useful means of ensuring that newly taught phonetic level

skills are transferred to phonology is to construct a series of word charts such as the one shown as Figure 9.6. Such charts should be constructed using words familiar to the child, and each should feature a given consonant in different vowel contexts. (Note the order in which the vowels are arranged.) In the example shown, the /ʃ/ is featured. By ensuring that the child is able to pronounce each word correctly, the teacher/clinician is providing both the child and herself with a substantial number of standard articula-

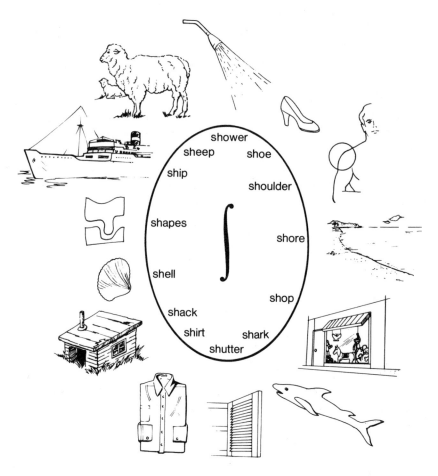

Figure 9.6

A word chart illustrating common vocabulary items beginning with /ʃ/. Words containing vowels having low formants are placed at the right; mid-frequency formants, low center; and high formants, at the left. Such words, when produced accurately, can be used as a guide to pronunciation of new vocabulary.

tions to which she can refer when teaching the pronunciation of new vocabulary. Children enjoy constructing such charts for themselves using some of the attractive colored pictures that are now widely available. Common words featuring /ʃ/ in other than initial positions, such as "fish" and "tissue," should also be featured in such charts.

Pronunciation of a word varies according to the stress it receives, its position in a sentence, and the number of words in the sentence. Teaching a child to produce sounds and then to use them in words is, therefore, not enough. One must be concerned with the rhythm and rate of spoken language if it is to be intelligible. Take the word "into" as an example. On its own it is pronounced /ɪntu/. In a short phrase such as "into the room," even when said quite slowly, the last vowel tends to be neutralized and the word pronounced /ɪntə/. Furthermore, the longer the phrase or sentence in which it is said, the shorter the word and all of its elements have to become. The reader may verify this by saying the word on its own and then in the sentence, "We went into that when we were at school." Consideration of these points indicates that beyond simple phonetic and phonologic level teaching lies a profound need for instruction in fluency (see D. Ling, 1976, pp. 215–216).

ANNOTATED BIBLIOGRAPHY

Calvert, D. R., and Silverman, S. R.   *Speech and Deafness.* Washington, D.C.: A.G. Bell Association for the Deaf, 1975.
This book provides an objective discussion of the major methodologies of speech teaching up to 1975, and in doing so places them in perspective. This is one of the most important texts on the topic published during this century and is strongly recommended for all concerned with the development of speech in hearing-impaired children.

Ling, D.   *Speech and the Hearing-Impaired Child: Theory and Practice.* Washington, D.C.: A.G. Bell Association for the Deaf, 1976. (See Annotated Bibliography for Chapter 4.)

Vorce, E.   *Teaching Speech to Deaf Children.* Washington, D.C.: A.G. Bell Association for the Deaf, 1974.

Written by a highly respected, master teacher, this text describes the speech teaching program in operation at the Lexington School for the Deaf, New York. It is easy to read and is recommended reading for students, teacher/clinicians, and administrators.

10. Parent-Infant Communication:

The Prelude to Spoken Language
Development in Normal-Hearing
and Hearing-Impaired Children

From the first days of life, the normal infant is capable of receiving information through his senses. He hears sounds and voices, receives visual impressions, is aware of touch, movement, and vibration, and has sensations of smell, taste, warmth, cold, and pain. At first, his reactions are mainly automatic and reflex in nature. For example, he startles or cries at very loud sounds, bright lights, and painful stimuli.

Normal Parent-Infant Interaction

The newborn infant spends much of his time asleep. When he wakes, he usually cries and is picked up, fed, bathed, and returned to his crib. He is quietly alert for brief periods only. Because his needs are well-known and are few in number, he does not require a complex communication system. Since he is usually cared for according to some sort of schedule, his needs are generally anticipated. When he cries, his mother usually responds. When her actions satisfy his needs, he stops crying and may either fall asleep or lie quietly, looking directly into her eyes. She will return his gaze. A rudimentary system of communication is at work.

Although a mother's elaborate verbal system of communication cannot possibly be understood and used by her infant, she does

180

not abandon it. Instead she accompanies her words with actions, looks, and varying tones of voice. She talks to him while she smiles, pats him, rocks him, bathes, diapers, and feeds him. The infant soon becomes active in seeking stimulation from his environment, and his potential for communication increases. He coos as well as cries, he lifts his head up, he looks intently at faces, his grasp becomes stronger, he kicks vigorously. He becomes quiet and still when he hears music or singing, or when someone speaks to him. The manner in which a baby acts and reacts can just as readily influence the people around him as they can him.

Vocal Communication in the First Months of Life

For most of the first year, the infant has to rely on crying as his only means of gaining attention when no one is nearby. Few mothers feel comfortable if they ignore their infants' crying. A mother becomes disturbed if her infant cries a great deal and she is unable to soothe him. However, she does not necessarily feel that a baby should be picked up or attended to, the instant he cries. The quality of the infant's cry will usually determine her reaction. Whimpering or fake crying will likely be ignored. Prolonged crying or a series of sharp, loud cries will usually secure a response. Until he is able to talk, the cause of his distress has to be discovered by his mother.

During the first months of life, the infant's vocalization is limited both in quantity and quality. He makes high-pitched squeaky sounds and throaty gurgles, all of which he can feel as well as hear. The sounds uttered by an infant are to some extent determined by his position. As he lies on his back, opens his mouth and vocalizes, an [æ]-like sound is emitted. He may produce something that sounds like a [g] through the contact of his tongue against the back of his palate. The infant has little or no control over the sounds he produces. The fact that an infant makes non-crying vocal sounds encourages his mother and those around him to talk to him. An even greater stimulus for interaction appears in the form of the infant's smile.

The Smile as a Base for Early Communication

Infants usually begin to smile when they are about four weeks old. The infant will smile at any face (or anything resembling a face), especially if the "face" smiles, moves, and talks. The eyes are the focus of the infant's attention. He gazes directly at the eyes and smiles. Eye contact and smiling are particularly important in establishing communication. As soon as he is able to smile, the infant becomes markedly more able to engage the attention of others around him. Few adults or children can resist smiling and talking in response. Mothers, fathers, brothers and sisters, strange adults, and children are easily enticed to interact with a smiling infant. Family members may vie with one another in eliciting his smile. The infant now has access to rich sources of interesting and varied stimulation.

How do people interact with a baby who is unable to talk? Sometimes sounds similar to his own are offered, and these are responded to with gurgles of delight. More often, spoken language is used. In speaking to the infant, the mother may raise the pitch of her voice closer to that of the infant's. His mother might say, "What do you want to tell me?" "Did you like your bottle, then?" She will pause between questions, smiling and making eye contact with her infant, waiting for him to make a response. In doing so, she is following normal conversational practice. If the infant responds by making any kind of vocalization, by smiling or moving his limbs about, his mother is likely to continue the conversation. If the infant remains completely unresponsive, she may persist in attempting to elicit a reaction, perhaps by tickling him. If she remains unsuccessful, she is likely to excuse him, perhaps saying, "Oh dear, you're too tired to talk now. Never mind." He will probably then be put back in his crib. An infant who rarely smiles is likely to receive little more than the minimum attention required for his physical care.

The infant of 3 to 6 months spends an increasing amount of time awake, and his mother tries out various ways to keep him happy and amused. He likes rattles, squeakers, and musical toys, but can manipulate few of them and when he drops something, he is unable to retrieve it. Most of all, he enjoys human contact. However, after some social stimulation, the young baby will usually be happy to be put in his crib. Left to himself, he is likely to continue cooing and vocalizing. He begins to experiment with his voice. He extends the range of vowel sounds that he produces. He makes sounds which are loud or quiet, high or low pitched, long or short, one at a time or in sequences. These infant sounds are hard to describe. Mothers may say their baby *"oohs* and *ahs."* The sounds are also hard to transcribe phonetically as they don't correspond exactly with the speech sounds made by adults. As the baby spends more time vocalizing, he almost inevitably increases the variety of sounds he produces. Talking, smiling, tickling, and playing with a baby are effective ways to increase the amount of time he spends in vocalizing.

Communication With Infants and Toddlers

By the age of 6 months, most babies can sit up with support and thus have a much better view of the world around them. They don't particularly like being left alone for long periods when they are awake. They enjoy being with people, family, friends and strangers alike. The 6- to 7-month-old baby usually turns around when his name is called or when he hears familiar or unfamiliar sounds. He laughs aloud and shouts to attract attention. He stretches his arms to be picked up. The first teeth usually begin to push through the gums and, as the baby feels the discomfort, he chews on hard objects and makes sounds such as [ana], [aja], [adada] and [amama]. The latter syllables are quickly picked up and imitated back to him by his parents.

Between 6 and 9 months, the baby extends his vocal repertoire. He will often imitate his own babbling sounds when those are spoken to him by his parents, but is quite unlikely to imitate syllables that are not part of his repertoire. The infant who spends a lot of time vocalizing will produce many different vowels and consonants in syllables. His sounds have increasing resemblance to those appearing in the speech he hears around him. He is gradually developing control over his vocal musculature and is integrating what he hears with what he says and what others say.

Between 9 months and a year, some parents report that their babies babble less than previously. The baby's attention may be greatly taken up by physical activity. As he learns to crawl, to pull himself to his feet and to take his first steps, he gives his attention to mastering these skills. His greater locomotor ability enables him to explore his environment, giving him access to a wide range of new and interesting experiences. He rarely wishes to remain still.

Not being able to talk hardly seems to hamper communication. The baby can babble, shout, laugh, smile, hold his arms up when he wants to be picked up, and shake his head to indicate he doesn't want something. He points at things he likes. When all else fails, he may cry and his mother usually manages to figure out what it is he wants.

During all of this time, the baby's mother has continued to talk to him while she cares for him. She washes, feeds, changes and dresses him. She also entertains him with toys and games. She continues to talk to him because he seems to listen and pay attention, often looking right into her eyes. She talks about what she is doing as she is doing it. She asks if he wants some milk as she is offering it to him. She points out what he can see and tells him about it. For example, "See the doggy. The dog goes bow-wow." She asks him questions such as "Where's Daddy?" and if he does not respond, or simply repeats "dada," she answers for him, pointing, "There he is. There's Daddy."

Before the baby can understand his mother's words, he interprets the situation from various angles. He utilizes cues from his previous experience of the situation and from what he can see and hear. For example, he will react to his mother's tone of voice and facial expression. If she shouts "No," he is likely to stop his actions immediately and perhaps cry. If, on the other hand, she says "No-no" in a pleasant voice while smiling, he is likely to suppose that what he is about to do is permitted, or perhaps that it is all part of a game.

As the baby grows older, his immediate wants become more specific, while the range of alternative desires becomes more extensive. His mother may be at a loss to know how to satisfy his needs. When he is thirsty, he may want juice, not water or milk. The ability to name what he wants offers a practical advantage and any attempts at word approximation, such as "oo" for "juice" will be quickly reinforced.

During his second year, the toddler with normal hearing switches increasingly from vocal to verbal communication. Nonverbal modes such as eye contact and facial expression, body posture, action and gesture come to be used as supplements, rather than alternatives to verbal expression. Communication development is markedly different for the infant born with impaired hearing.

The Untreated Hearing-Impaired Infant and His Parents

Parents rarely suspect hearing impairment at or soon after birth unless there is some special reason—such as deafness in another family member, maternal rubella, or complications at birth. In the majority of cases, the infant is examined and proclaimed "normal" before being released from the hospital. His parents will therefore tend to presume that the infant's hearing is normal, until they have evidence to the contrary. Their expectations about how he ought to respond to sound are likely to be rather vague because landmarks in the development of listening skills are not common knowledge.

During the first year of life, as we mentioned earlier, the mother accepts the burden of communication and interprets the vocal and nonverbal cues offered by the infant. The severely or profoundly hearing-impaired infant will communicate by crying, vocalizing, smiling, making eye contact, moving his arms and legs. He may be so alert to his visual environment that his unawareness of sound passes unnoticed. If the infant's failure to respond to sound is remarked on, it might not at first be attributed to hearing impairment. Lack of interest, immaturity, or because he is "so accustomed to noise that he ignores it" may be advanced as reasons for lack of response. He may be characterized as a quiet, good baby who sleeps a great deal and is not disturbed by noise. As he grows older, the infant's abnormal responses to sound will become increasingly obvious when compared with the responses of other infants. Since he cannot hear he does not startle to loud, unexpected sounds, nor is he soothed by his mother's voice, but only by her appearing within his view. He does not show any interest in noises which are produced by people or objects outside his visual field.

For the first few months of life, even though he is unable to hear his own voice, the hearing-impaired infant cries and vocalizes in much the same way as the normal infant. However, as he grows older, his repertoire tends to remain restricted both with respect to quantity and quality, and he may not develop syllabic babble. By the end of the first year, his vocalization may be reduced to sounds he can feel—high-pitched squeaks and guttural sounds, similar to those of a one-month-old. Since he cannot hear the sounds he makes, he fails to develop auditory feedback. He cannot match the sounds he produces on one occasion with those he produces a little later, or with those made by others. He does not discover for himself how to produce sounds that are loud or quiet, high or low, long or short. He does not develop control over his voice, his breathing, or his articulation.

In the absence of habilitative treatment for the child and guidance for his parents, communication between them becomes increasingly difficult. The normal child begins to give some evidence of understanding what is said, albeit by the help of nonverbal cues. The untreated hearing-impaired child makes no attempt to listen to what is said and his behavior may become difficult to manage. Since he does not understand the spoken word, he has to rely heavily on eye contact, facial expression, action and gesture, together with his interpretation of the ongoing situation and his past experience. As his parents become aware, consciously or subconsciously, of his inability to understand speech, they will talk less to him since there appears to be little point in doing so. They will tend to rely increasingly on nonverbal modes of communication. Yet, like his hearing counterpart, the hearing-impaired child's desires become more and more complex and difficult to achieve through nonverbal means. Frustration is almost inevitable, and temper tantrums may easily become a fairly permanent feature of his behavior instead of merely a passing phase. If neither parent nor child has received help before he is 3 years old, he is likely to become mute, apart from laughing, crying, and screaming. His parents are likely to adopt defensive strategies in dealing with him. They may be unable to leave him in the care of a sitter. Although by age 3 or 4 he should be enjoying playing with his peers, problems are likely to arise because of his inability either to talk or to understand what is being said. He may easily become a loner either because he is rejected on account of aggressive behavior such as fighting, grabbing and pushing, or because he withdraws into his own world.

Despite his inability to acquire spoken language, the hearing-impaired child is capable of learning a great deal through senses other than audition. He perceives and appreciates the orderly routines of his daily life. He achieves a feeling of security from a knowledge of what happens and where things belong. He develops extreme visual alertness. He scans his environment, checks for familiarity, and quickly notes changes, even small ones. His visual memory for places and events may surprise his family. His evident intelligent behavior may lead to his hearing impairment not being diagnosed by doctors who see him only in a clinic, and the reason for his lack of language may be sought elsewhere.

The continuing refusal of the family practitioner or pediatrician to determine whether or not parental suspicion of hearing impairment is valid may seriously jeopardize the chances of a successful outcome. Audiologists and teachers, as well as doctors, need to listen when parents report on communication problems either initially or in later years. Frequently, increased hearing impairment is first spotted by parents in the course of daily interaction. Follow-up testing should reveal the cause, perhaps a middle-ear problem or a progressive loss.

Effects of Mild and Moderate Hearing Impairments on Communication

Even a mild to moderate hearing impairment such as that associated with frequent ear infections can result in delayed speech and language development. The effects become increasingly severe if the impairment continues throughout the second and third years of life since the child spends a great deal of time at some distance from those speaking to him.

The child who has good hearing for low-frequency sounds but poor hearing for the high-frequency consonants is neither normal nor similar to a profoundly hearing-impaired infant in developing communication skills. Infants who are capable of hearing their own voices and those of others, without amplification, are likely to follow the normal steps of early auditory and vocal development. In the first months of life, adequate auditory stimulation is available in that the infant with a moderate or high-frequency hearing impairment can hear his mother since she talks to him principally when holding him or bending over his crib. She is speaking very close to his ear, thus providing him with a high level of sound. Syllabic babble may be somewhat delayed and is unlikely to be abundant and varied, but may still be sufficient to be considered within normal limits.

The child with a moderate or high-tone loss may be delayed in learning to understand what is said to him. His vocabulary of spoken words is likely to be acquired slowly and his attempts at sentence construction are likely to result in jargon incomprehensible to others. Because such children are demonstrably capable of hearing a wide variety of sounds, their speech and language deficiencies may be attributed to slowness rather than to hearing impairment. They may be variously described as inconsistent in responding to sound, listening only when they want to, being stubborn, inattentive or lazy, or absorbed in their own interests.

Although the provision of appropriate hearing aids will give access to much clearer and more complete auditory patterns, the effects of the period of language deprivation are not instantly erased. Contrary to what the parents might expect, the child's speech and language do not automatically become normal. Parents and child should be enrolled in a habilitation program which includes counseling about the psychological effects of hearing impairment as well as techniques in the use of hearing and the enrichment of language.

The Hearing-Impaired Infant With Additional Problems

Hearing impairment is sometimes discovered early in life following initial concern with cataracts, heart defect, or cerebral palsy. Early identification, however, may create psychological problems for the parents. Mother-infant communication is likely to follow a somewhat different path when the newborn infant requires immediate placement in intensive care or is immediately noticed as having a defect. The shock of discovering that their infant is not perfect creates deep grief in the parents and may prevent them from interacting warmly and normally with the baby. If the infant's life is in danger, hearing impairment becomes a matter of secondary concern, and hopes regarding his long-term future development are shelved. When released from the hospital, a hearing-impaired infant who has had intensive care as a newborn is likely to be treated with special attention and, rather than being encouraged to explore his environment, his activities may be restricted to prevent further harm. Parental expectations may be altered. The child's needs may continue to be anticipated and supplied beyond the usual age for beginning verbal communication, and his motivation to develop it may consequently be reduced.

Two of the most serious additional handicaps are autism and blindness. Autistic traits such as avoiding eye contact, rejection of physical contact, rocking and head-banging impose severe strains on communication. Parents of hearing-impaired infants with such additional problems urgently require help. The combination of deafness and blindness is a formidable one. The untreated infant receives little or no information through either hearing or vision, and has incredibly restricted input from his environment. Communication is established, if at all, principally through touch. The senses of smell and taste are usually pressed into greater service. Unless greatly stimulated by others, the child will have difficulty in developing in cognitive areas. Extraordinary persistence in the child, his parents, and his teachers will be essential for developing what would otherwise be thought of as ordinary skills. Habilitation for multiply handicapped children depends on a concerted team effort.

The Hearing-Impaired Infant With Deaf Parents

Parents who are themselves deaf are likely to detect hearing impairment in their own infants with greater facility than the professionals. Their acute visual observations are a major asset.

The communication skills of the parents will influence the manner in which they interact with their infants. Regardless of whether they themselves communicate by spoken language or sign language, deaf parents are concerned that they be alerted to their infant's cry. A vocally operated flashing light is one solution. This permits mother and infant to establish a very basic communication system. Nonverbal modes such as eye contact, smiling, body contact and action will probably be used even more extensively than normal. Deaf parents may make renewed attempts to find hearing aids which would allow them the pleasure of hearing their baby's coos and gurgles. They are often successful in this, since many modern hearing aids are superior to the models that were formerly available. The birth of a hearing-impaired child to deaf parents may be a cause of some disappointment, but does not create fear and panic in such parents since deafness is a familiar and ever-present part of their daily lives. Such acceptance provides a firm base for communication.

Habilitation for such an infant will depend on the choice of the parents. In the event that the parents communicate with one another by sign language, they themselves will be the child's natural teachers. For those who wish their child to develop oral communication skills, problems abound, in that the infant of deaf parents has less access to normal patterns of spoken language. However, the assistance of relatives and friends can be secured. This could also be essential in the case of any normal-hearing infants they might have.

Habilitation of the Hearing-Impaired Infant

The Diagnostic Period

If there is reason to suspect that the infant might be hearing-impaired, habilitative steps should be recommended to parents at the time of initial testing. Parents should talk quietly, but directly, into the baby's ear, as well as in a face-to-face situation. In this way it is possible for the child to hear at least something of his parents' voices, and to feel the varied breath flow of their speech against his cheek. From the first month or so of life, the parents can increase the quantity of the baby's vocalization by talking to him, smiling at him, tickling him, and mimicking his sounds. Should the infant be found to have normal hearing, no harm has been done. Should the baby be hearing-impaired, no time has been lost in providing him with some auditory and tactile information about speech, and in reinforcing his own attempts at vocalizing.

The parents should also be informed of the range of possible responses made to sound by normal-hearing infants, and encouraged to observe the reactions of their own and other infants. This procedure helps parents to make their own judgments and match them with the outcome of diagnostic tests. Parents need to feel that the test results are valid; otherwise they will seek one professional opinion after another, until they find someone who will confirm their viewpoint or, alternatively, some one who will take the time to explain the nature of the tests and the implications of the diagnosis. Details on current diagnostic procedures are provided in Chapter 5.

A careful explanation of the child's problem may lead the parents to ask (rather than be told) whether a hearing aid might be helpful. A demonstration may offer some immediate evidence. Since the infant does not yet have his own earmolds, a stethoscope-style attachment can be used to permit him to receive sound amplified by means of a personal hearing aid. The parents should be asked to talk softly to their baby, close to the microphone of the aid, as the clinician rotates the volume control back and forth. Once again, the clinician has to explain what type of responses may reasonably be expected, since the parents may otherwise not be prepared to accept the clinician's judgment concerning the infant's responses. For example, the parents may consider that turning the head toward the source of sound is an acceptable response, whereas the clinician may be satisfied if the infant becomes quiet or still. Possible reasons for lack of response should also be discussed. The preparation of parents for probable reactions is especially beneficial when the baby has been fitted with his own personal hearing aids.

Hearing Aid Selection

As discussed in Chapter 6, the selection of hearing aids does not have to be postponed until a pure tone audiogram has been obtained. Reasonable estimates of gain, frequency range, tolerance levels, and maximum power output (SSPL 90) are sufficient. Audiologists may be afraid of fitting infants with high-gain hearing aids because of the possibility of exposing babies to excessive noise levels and further damaging their hearing. However, insufficient amplification also has serious consequences. The infant may be denied the opportunity to hear speech at optimal levels; he may merely be enabled to detect sounds, rather than to distinguish them clearly, with the result that progress in the acquisition of hearing, speech, and language skills is unnecessarily slow. The solution lies in the selection of hearing aids with adjustable controls for maximum power output, frequency range, and compression so that the settings can be altered in the course of ongoing assessment and habilitation.

Infants have particular need for amplification over the widest possible frequency range. During the first year or so of life, the suprasegmental aspects of spoken language are especially important. First of all, the infant can derive meaning from tone of voice and intonation patterns before he is able to do so from the phonetic or segmental aspects. Secondly, in order to develop an abundance of well-intonated vocalization, the infant needs to hear his own voice (F_0 in the region of 300 Hz) as well as that of his parents (F_0 around 80-150 Hz for males and 200-300 Hz for females). The inclusion of the low-frequency end of the spectrum should make it possible for hearing-impaired infants to develop and maintain natural voice quality. Such a requirement does not preclude the use of a frequency range extending well beyond 3000 Hz (say to 5000 or 6000 Hz) so that important phonemes such as [s] can be amplified and made audible and even discriminable to infants with sufficient residual hearing.

For practical reasons, we still generally prefer to fit children under the age of 3 with body rather than ear-level aids. Between the ages of 1 and 3 years, the child's behavior is unpredictable and he may lose an entire hearing aid, rather than just a mold and receiver. Loss of the ear-level aid is less likely to be detected soon enough to make discovery possible. The aid may be lost out of doors or flushed down a toilet. For infants, body aids with the microphone on the front of the aid are preferable to those with a top placement, where the microphone is vulnerable to spills and dirt. Infants as well as older children should have aids with a telecoil position to allow for use with a loop system, especially in the case of profound hearing impairment. Once the child is crawling or walking, he will spend more of his time at a considerable distance from his mother and, without the help of a loop or FM system, the child may not hear optimally. His progress in acquiring spoken language will therefore be unnecessarily slow.

How To Wear Body Aids

When body aids are selected for young children, we insist upon their being worn on top of their clothing so that the child has optimal opportunity to hear his own voice and the voices of others. To wear the aids under clothing is equivalent to increasing the child's hearing impairment. We have found it convenient to have the aids worn in a sturdy harness of soft leather. The leather which covers the microphone is perforated. Adjustable straps allow for the harness to be worn comfortably on top of thin or thick clothing. For Canadian winters, mothers sew pockets onto their children's snowsuits. Parents and clinicians have ready access to aids which are worn on top of outer clothing. We do not attempt to fit body aids on a young child without having the harness available. Once the aids have been adjusted they can be put into the pockets of the harness, and the child can be permitted freedom of movement.

Fitting the Hearing Aids

Success in initial fitting of hearing aids to infants and young children depends on the attitudes of the parents and clinicians. If the clinician is uncertain as to whether hearing aids can be of help to a particular child, or if she expresses doubt—either spoken or unspoken—as to whether the child will keep the molds in his ears, the chances are that such feelings will be communicated to the parents. Our approach is one of optimism. Almost all hearing-impaired infants and young children have some hearing and, when such hearing is used from infancy, habilitation has a better chance of success than when hearing aids are introduced at a later stage.

Babies enjoy being able to hear. Hearing aids should not, therefore, be thought of as nasty medicine which must be taken in order to cure an illness. Modern-day infants with severe or profound hearing impairment are fortunate indeed compared with those born 20 or 30 years ago, when suitable hearing aids were not available. A positive attitude should be conveyed by the teacher/clinician to the parents. Parents, in turn, should be helped to realize that they should try to smile rather than frown while putting the earmolds in the baby's ears. From the very beginning, the mold should be fitted into the baby's ear before switching the aid on. This procedure avoids unnecessary acoustic howl; more important, when this procedure is followed each time the aids are put on, it helps draw the infant's attention to the contrast between absence and presence of sound. The parent or clinician talks to the child: "Here's your hearing aid. Let's put the mold in your ear. Oh dear, I can't get it in. In it goes. Let's switch it on. Can you hear me now? Bababa, booboobooo." The baby is then encouraged to take his turn in conversation. Should he chance to vocalize at this point and hear his own voice, he may be quite surprised. A brief vocal interchange between parent and child may ensue. Otherwise, the baby's mother or father should be encouraged to talk softly to him, close to the microphone of his aids, smiling and pausing every now and then, trying to elicit some vocalization. If the baby vocalizes, his own sounds should be mimicked.

When the infant pulls out an earmold, his mother should be encouraged to replace it gently but firmly, smile and talk to him, and then distract his attention. For the first few days, the baby or young child will require supervision while he is wearing his aids; he may keep trying to remove the molds, much as he might struggle to remove mittens or a hat. A baby is likely to stop trying to remove his molds as soon as he becomes aware of sound and can enjoy the increased experiences available. Full-time usage of aids can usually be established within a week.

Reactions to the Hearing Aids

Parents are often puzzled by their child's behavior in the first stage of hearing aid use. They may report that he is quiet when wearing the aids, and noisy when they are removed. A reasonable explanation would seem to be that while he is wearing his aids he becomes aware of many of the sounds in his environment and stops vocalizing in order to listen. When the aids are removed, he may vocalize or create a lot of noise in order to try and provide himself with auditory stimulation. Parents who have not been warned of the possibility of such reactions may quickly conclude that the hearing aids are of little help. We have found it useful to provide parents with a list of reactions and responses frequently observed in the early stages of hearing aid use (see A. H. Ling, 1977).

The teacher/clinician should telephone the parents within one or two days of fitting the aid to check on progress, to offer further suggestions, support, and encouragement, and to answer questions. It is particularly helpful to parents if the teacher/clinician indicates that they are free to call her at anytime should they be worried. By making herself available in this way, the teacher/clinician assures the parents that she cares about their difficulties outside the clinic and helps to establish a good relationship which is crucial to the success of early habilitative work.

Testing the Aids

Parents should be encouraged to listen carefully to their children's aids while they are new, so that they can become alert to deterioration of the quality or clarity of amplified speech. In addition to a thorough check at the end of each day, parents of babies and young children should check the aids quickly, in the morning (and after naps), in front of the child using the Five-Sound-Test (see Chapter 6). The conscientious practice of this routine over a period of several months by one young mother led to her hearing-impaired baby spontaneously saying "oo-ah-ee" as her aids were put on.

Development of Listening Skills

From the moment when hearing aids are fitted, the infant or young child should be introduced to sounds which are likely to interest him and should be reinforced for attending or responding to them. Parents therefore have to be helped to discover what kinds of experiences their baby would enjoy, and also what constitutes a response.

A common viewpoint has been that the hearing-impaired child should be bombarded or bathed with sound, to make up for any auditory deprivation he may have suffered. Some parents have thought that it would be helpful for the child to watch a lot of TV or to listen to the stereo. This approach is most often followed by, or recommended to, parents who are not fluent speakers of the language the child is to learn. One consequence of providing continual auditory stimulation which is not meaningful to the child, is that he will soon come to ignore sound. Another consequence is that he will have difficulty hearing his own voice against the background of noise and will probably be discouraged from experimenting vocally.

For reasons of tradition, audiologists may suggest that nonverbal sounds such as bells, rattles, whistles, and drums should be used. Certainly, infants enjoy rattles and squeaker toys, especially when they can manipulate them themselves. Older babies enjoy playing with saucepans. The guiding principle should be that the child enjoys the experience, rather than that he be trained to respond each time he hears a drum or whistle. Sounds which are a regular feature of the child's environment should be drawn to his attention. The 6-month-old will be excited by the barking of the family pet. He will like the sound and movement of airplanes and helicopters and will soon learn to look up for them.

Much of the difficulty encountered by teacher/clinicians in trying to figure out appropriate auditory experiences for infants has been due to (1) a lack of realization that the sounds which are most absorbing to a normal-hearing infant are the sounds of speech, and (2) the belief that little of human speech could be made audible to a baby with a profound hearing impairment. The preceding chapters have shown what aspects of speech should be audible to children with different degrees of hearing impairment. This knowledge should provide teacher/clinicians with the confidence that listening to speech is indeed the most crucial auditory experience for the hearing-impaired infant. It seems that the infant brain is tuned to the early processing of speech and that the development of spoken language is facilitated when audition is utilized to the maximum.

Listening and Vocalizing

The development of listening skills should be intimately related to expanding the baby's vocal repertoire. Opportunities for listening and vocalizing can easily be fitted into the daily routine of child care. The baby's mother should try to attract his attention through audition by calling his name, "Hi Johnny. Mommy's coming," before she appears in his visual field. She should smile and talk to him, then pause to give him a chance to vocalize before she picks him up. She can talk softly against his cheek as she carries him, for his attention does not always have to be on her face before she speaks. She can talk to him while she bathes or diapers him, remembering to speak right into his ear if he is not wearing his aids. She may be quiet while she feeds him, but talk as she burps him. When the baby is happy and content, he will usually vocalize spontaneously, or can easily be encouraged to do so. This is the time to indulge in vocal games, following the baby's lead where possible. The more the baby can be encouraged to vocalize, the more likely he will retain good voice quality, and the greater variety of sounds he will produce. As with the normal-hearing baby, the sounds produced by the hearing-impaired baby are not at first under conscious control. However, the more he vocalizes, the more he becomes aware of his own voice (i.e., develops auditory feedback). Soon he is able to produce certain sounds, or aspects of sounds, deliberately. As was explained in earlier chapters, such feedforward control is essential for fluent speech.

As soon as the baby is accustomed to wearing his aids, it may be worthwhile to leave them on when he is put down for a nap. Babies often engage in a prolonged period of vocalizing and babbling before falling asleep. If the room is quiet and only dimly lit, the baby's attention is even more likely to focus upon auditory-vocal activity. Hearing-impaired babies benefit from this type of self-directed experience.

No formal speech training is envisaged with the hearing-impaired infant. The skillful teacher/clinician, however, can demonstrate to the parents how they can help their baby explore his vocal capacities. The stages of speech development proposed for the hearing-impaired child are valid for the infant, but different strategies will need to be used. Parents can offer their baby a variety of vocal patterns as models. The baby should be comfortably held on one's lap, in a face-to-face position. Choosing one of the vowels used by the baby, his mother (or father) might produce it in a series of short, staccato bursts, followed by a prolonged vowel; or a series of quiet vowels followed by a loud one; or an ascending or descending series. The vocal activity might be accompanied by physical activity and vivid facial expression. Babies delight in such stimulation and may want to touch the mouths and faces of those producing the sounds. Baby's repertoire will gradually become more extensive as a result of this type of activity.

Parents wishing to introduce vowel sounds not present in the infant's repertoire should try those which are adjacent to vowels already produced, moving from center to front or center to back vowels. Alternatively, for the baby who enjoys putting his fingers in his mother's mouth, contrasts such as "oo-ee" and "ee-oo" would provide strong tactile patterns. After several months of this type of vocal play, syllabic babble such as [adada] will appear unexpectedly, creating great joy and excitement. The parents should follow the baby's lead and imitate his patterns, rather than continually presenting new models which may be beyond his capability. The key notion is one of play and fun.

For the child who is more than a year old, such vocal play may be enjoyed in the context of somewhat rougher physical play with Dad, or as part of a pre-bedtime interchange. It may be introduced in a game involving toy animals and vehicles with which different patterns of sound can be associated.

Listening to Language

A major portion of the normal infant's auditory experience consists of spoken language. If the hearing-impaired infant is to learn to talk, he must have comparable opportunities. He can learn to make the necessary associations between spoken patterns and their intended meanings. He, too, can use cues from the situation, from his mother's tone of voice and facial expression. Because the auditory patterns he receives are often distorted or incomplete, however, he requires more frequent exposure in order to learn. The repetitive nature of the baby's daily routine and his dependence on adults provide ample opportunity for such exposure. Short phrases commenting on the situations rather than repeated naming of objects, should be used, and the mother should try to sense what aspect of the situation is the focus of the baby's attention at that moment and talk accordingly.

Impoverished input is often the result of the parents' failure to understand how speech and language normally develop. They may call their child's name over and over again, even when the child has responded once or twice. Their sole purpose seems to be one of determining whether or not he can hear it. This is counter-productive, as the child will soon learn to ignore sound. Such parents need to be helped to understand normal development and particularly to accept that, like the normal-hearing child, the hearing-impaired child requires a period of listening and babbling before he can be expected to understand and use spoken language.

A tactic that many workers have found helpful is to explain the concept that a baby's "hearing age" should be calculated from the time when full-time hearing aid use is established. Thus, initial responses to amplified sound would be similar to those of a new-born baby. This concept should not, however, be interpreted literally. A hearing-impaired baby fitted with hearing aids is not endowed with the auditory capacities of a normal-hearing new-born infant. Hearing aids only partially compensate for the hearing impairment. The effects of three months' hearing aid use are not likely to be equivalent for children with moderate, severe, and profound hearing impairment. Some of the other factors involved are the age from which aids are worn on a full-time basis, the quantity and quality of listening experience, and, of course, whether or not the hearing aids are appropriate.

Some parents and teacher/clinicians may be uncertain about the type of vocabulary and phrases which are suitable for use with a hearing-impaired baby. The best guide is to follow the needs and interests of the child. A list of questions and phrases commonly used by mothers to their normal-hearing babies, and consequently among those first understood, is included as an appendix to this chapter. This list has been found useful by mothers of hearing-impaired babies, especially in families where English is not the native language.

Appropriate social behavior can be encouraged. From about 10 months, the hearing-impaired baby can be shown how to wave bye-bye. At first, his mother can help him move his hand while she says "Bye-bye. Wave bye-bye" with a characteristic sing-song intonation pattern. Soon the baby learns to wave when someone is leaving the room. Later he responds to the intonation pattern and eventually the phonetic (or auditory-visual) pattern of the words, without the help of situational cues.

Songs and rhymes should be included for the baby's entertainment. In addition to being a part of our culture, they provide much greater pitch and intonation contrasts than does conversation. The hearing-impaired baby will enjoy being rocked to and fro to the rhyme "Hush-a-bye baby" and will soon anticipate being "dropped" when the singer reaches "down will go baby, cradle and all."

Vocal Communication

Vocal communication should be developed in the hearing-impaired child as a forerunner to verbal communication. While normal use of nonverbal modes such as eye contact, facial expression, gesture, and body posture is desirable, parents should be wary of relying exclusively on them. From the beginning of habilitation, the baby should be reinforced for vocalizing in response to speech. By the age of 8 or 9 months, the baby can be encouraged to use a loud voice as a means of attracting attention. When the baby happens to use a loud voice, his mother should react with surprise, looking up from what she is doing, or coming from another room and saying, "Mommy heard you calling. What do you want?" Mother can initiate games of "peek-a-boo" or "hide-and-seek" involving an older child who can call "John-ny. Mommy. Where are you?" getting a reply such as "Cuckoo. Hi there. Here I am." Somewhat exaggerated intonation patterns should be used.

The hearing-impaired child of a year or more will tend to communicate by tugging, pointing, gesturing, and even screaming or having a temper tantrum, unless he is otherwise trained. It is crucial that he behave in ways considered appropriate for his age. Firm and consistent handling is required and will provide the hearing-impaired child with the comfort and security of knowing what is expected of him.

Simple reinforcement techniques can be used to foster vocal communication until such time as the child has some word approximations. If a mother responds quickly to her child's vocal efforts, and consistently ignores physical actions, she will find that her message is understood. Once again, an older brother or sister can act as a model. He may say, "Come on, Mommy." Alternatively, the mother can ask, "What do you want? . . . Do you want Mommy to come? . . . Tell Mommy, Get up." She should pause between each question, and if the child vocalizes, perhaps "uh," she says "Okay, Mommy's getting up. Let's see what you want."

The hearing-impaired child who vocalizes extensively in play can be expected to use varied intonation patterns, and angry and happy tones of voice in communicating his needs. Greetings such as "hi" and "bye" and expressions such as "ow!" and "oh-oh" are easily learned. As the child begins to give evidence of understanding something of what is said and vocalizes abundantly for pleasure, he will begin to use some word approximations. As with the normal-hearing child, one never can tell what words will be the first used by the hearing-impaired child.

From Vocal to Verbal Communication

For a child's utterance to be accepted as a word approximation, it must have something in common with the adult form. Thus "oo" would be an approximation for "shoe" or "juice," whereas "eh" or "uh" would not. If the hearing-impaired child regularly says "ba" when he means "come," and the adult responds by coming, the child is reinforced in his use of "ba." If this process is allowed to persist, the hearing-impaired child might develop such an original lexicon that only his mother understands him. When the child says "ba," showing by action or gesture that he wishes his mother to come, she should pretend she does not understand. She should repeat the syllable with a frowning expression, "Ba? Ba? What do you want? Do you want Mommy to come? You tell Mommy, come." Imitation is not forced, but hopefully the child will reproduce at least the vowel. In this way the child is helped to become aware of the correspondence of particular auditory/articulatory sequences and their generally accepted meanings. His attention is focused on the similarities and differences of various sound patterns. Vocal imitation helps to establish auditory/articulatory coding of differentiated patterns in memory. The child's ability to produce a recognizable approximation of a word undoubtedly affects the rapidity with which his spoken vocabulary grows.

The hearing-impaired child should be reinforced for his early approximations to phrases such as "all-gone," "put-it-back," "there-it-is," and "shut-the-door." Teacher/clinicians and parents should make no attempt to segment those units into separate words and have the child attempt to imitate them one by one. These phrases are normally learned as units and segmented only at a later date.

Assessing Progress

Assessment forms a crucial part of any habilitation program. It offers a firm base for planning and allows for the measurement of the effectiveness of intervention. Some types of tests (for example, a neurological examination) are administered only once if there are no negative findings. Others, such as otologic, audiologic, and developmental (psychological) tests, are undertaken periodically, or when indicated. Yet others may be given as part of a research study. Audio and video tape recordings are utilized to trace speech, language, and communication development.

Habilitation is facilitated by frequent monitoring of the child's status in the areas of most concern. Such monitoring is helpful not only to the teacher/clinician in planning individual programs, but also to the parents in enabling them to become aware of the many small steps which have to be taken en route to a long-term goal. It can be therapeutic for them to record their child's development.

The faster the child progresses, the easier it will be for the parents to come to grips with the permanence of the hearing impairment, and the more they will be able to participate in the habilitation program. Anxiety for the child's future often tends to paralyze parents. They may worry endlessly, becoming increasingly depressed and failing to interact warmly and joyfully with their hearing-impaired baby. Hope for the child's future leads to positive action.

A. Ling has prepared *Schedules of Development in Audition, Speech, Language and Communication* for this purpose. The parent and teacher/clinician should each have his or her own copy. The Schedules are suitable for infants and preschool children, regardless of the degree of hearing impairment, and of the age at which training begins. The professional should help the parent establish what skills the baby already has, and then both should discuss how succeeding steps in each schedule might be achieved. No promises for the long-term future can reasonably be made since many factors are involved, but short-term plans can be put forward.

The extent of the child's hearing impairment and the age at which habilitation is begun will markedly affect the level at which the child commences. The child's present chronological age and his levels of development in locomotor, personal-social, and hand-eye coordination will also influence the type of strategies which can be used to facilitate verbal communication in the context of healthy overall growth. A baby with limited hearing will require more visual input than one with good residual hearing. A 2-year-old child newly fitted with hearing aids will require different types of activity to increase the quantity of vocalization than would a 6-month-old.

A knowledge of normal infant development is essential as a basis for planning early habilitative work with hearing-impaired infants. The professional also needs to know something of the effects of such problems as autism, visual defects, cerebral palsy, and mental retardation since these may occur in combination with hearing impairment. The ideal way to learn about early childhood, and what is involved in being a parent 24 hours a day, is to have children of one's own. It is a humbling experience. It is very easy for a non-parent to dispense free advice on child raising. Direct experience in caring for children on a round-the-clock basis could be obtained by offering to look after a neighbor's family for a weekend. Students would learn a great deal from daytime and evening babysitting with various families, some with normal-hearing and others with hearing-impaired children. Even those who have experienced the joys and worries of parenthood cannot fully appreciate the grief of discovering that one's child has a serious handicap or disability of a permanent nature, a handicap with which one is unfamiliar and for which one is unprepared.

Benefits of Early Intervention

When hearing impairment is diagnosed before the age of 6 months, treatment can be habilitative rather than remedial, since it is possible to lay the foundations for verbal learning during the period when they normally occur. The earlier in life that an infant is able to hear his own and others' voices (albeit imperfectly), the less will be the effects of auditory deprivation, and the less he will turn to his other senses for information that is normally obtained through hearing.

Hearing and speech skills can be fostered more readily when they are developed in tune with the child's locomotor, personal-social, and cognitive development. The 3-month-old hearing-impaired baby, because he smiles and coos in the normal way, is able to elicit abundant input from surrounding adults. The baby is reinforced for vocalizing, and increases the amount of time he spends vocalizing. Because the baby responds to their talking, the adults, in turn, are reinforced and spend more time amusing the baby. The hearing-impaired baby who is fitted with appropriate aids in the early months of life benefits from having a prolonged period during which to develop auditory-vocal skills, without his parents worrying that he is not yet showing signs of understanding speech or beginning to talk. Furthermore, the baby does not have too many enticing activities to distract him from vocal play.

This is not the case toward the end of the first year, when he will be busy learning how to crawl and walk. As soon as he is mobile, there is so much to explore. It clearly requires greater ingenuity and persistence on the part of the mother to ensure that the hearing-impaired toddler has sufficient opportunity to develop auditory-vocal skills and to try to grasp the meanings of spoken language at the same time. The hearing-impaired child who has had an early start will have a basic phonetic repertoire on which to build language, although it will probably be less extensive than that of the child with normal hearing.

When habilitation begins early, the teacher/clinician can depend to a great extent on the normal intuitive reactions of parents to their infants. The parents are likely to realize that they are the most important people in their baby's life, and they are not likely to hand over responsibility for his upbringing to someone else. The situation is quite different for parents who do not receive guidance at an early stage and who experience distress and failure. They may have given up hope.

ANNOTATED BIBLIOGRAPHY

Brazelton, T. B.   *Infants and Mothers.* New York: Dell Publishing Co., 1969.
This is a beautifully illustrated, easy to read book, written by a pediatrician. He traces the development of three infants—a very active, a moderately active, and a quiet baby—during the first year of life, revealing their individuality and describing their interaction with their mothers. Professionals involved in parent-infant work will find it helpful as will young mothers themselves.

Freeman, P.   *Understanding the Deaf-Blind Child.* London, Eng.: Wm. Heinemann Medical Books, 1975.
Written by the mother of a slow-developing, deaf-blind Rubella child, this book will be appreciated by parents and teacher/clinicians for the insight it provides, as well as for the wealth of practical suggestions. Awarded an M.B.E. for her work, Mrs. Freeman writes not only from experiences with her own child and those of other parents belonging to the National Deaf/Blind and Rubella Children's Association which she founded, but also as a qualified teacher of multiply handicapped children.

Knobloch, H., and Pasamanick, B. (Eds.)   *Gesell and Armatru-da's Developmental Diagnosis* (3rd ed.). New York: Harper and Row, 1974.
Although hearing impairment receives scant treatment in this text, it will nevertheless be found useful by professionals working in the diagnosis of hearing impairment, and the early stages of habilitation. Chapter 18 provides an excellent discussion of Parent Management.

Leach, P.   *Babyhood.* New York: Alfred A. Knopf, 1976.
An informative and well-written book on the physical, emotional, and mental development of babies in the first two years of life. The author integrates knowledge gained from research. Of interest to professionals and parents alike.

Ling, A. H.   *Schedules of Development in Audition, Speech, Language and Communication for Hearing-Impaired Infants and Their Parents.* Washington, D.C.: The A. G. Bell Association for the Deaf, 1977.
A 15-page assessment guide and record for use by parents and teacher/clinicians.

Northcott, W. H. (Ed.)   *Curriculum Guide: Hearing-Impaired Children (0-3 years) and Their Parents.* Washington, D.C.: The A. G. Bell Association for the Deaf, (Rev. ed.), 1977.
This book contains a wealth of information on various aspects of a parent-infant program for hearing-impaired children. The accent is on parent participation in the development of listening and language skills. Behavioral objectives relating to normal hearing and normal behavior are provided, and various evaluation tools are described. Included are 31 appendices comprising record forms, check lists, etc. utilized by the authors.

Pushaw, D. R.   *Teach Your Child To Talk* (Rev. ed.) New York: CEBCO Standard Publishing, 1976.
This inexpensive paperback is written for parents to encourage them in developing speech and language skills in their children. The author traces development in six-month periods from birth to 2 years, and then in one-year periods to age 5. Included are questions for parents to answer at each stage in relation to their own child. Many activities are

suggested. The book is easy to read, and cartoon illustrations add to the informal way in which the information is presented. Helpful for parents, teacher/clinicians, and students training for parent-infant work.

Stream, R. W., and Stream, K. S.   Counseling the parents of the hearing-impaired child. In F. N. Martin (Ed.), *Pediatric Audiology.* Englewood Cliffs, N.J.: Prentice-Hall, Inc., 1978.
Essential reading for teacher/clinicians involved in diagnostic and habilitative work.

Vaughan, P. (Ed.)   *Learning To Listen.* Don Mills, Ontario: New Press, 1976.
A delightful little book written by parents for other parents of hearing-impaired children. It describes the use of an auditory approach to language learning and provides lots of practical suggestions for activities, procedures, games. Professionals also should read this book.

APPENDIX

Words, Phrases, and Questions Understood by Babies

Where's . . . . (own name)?
Where's Mommy?
Where's Daddy?
Where's . . . . (Brother/Sister)?

Show me your nose, eyes, hair, etc.
Where's your . . . . ?

Find your shoe, sock, coat, etc.
Give it to Mommy.
Take off your shoes.

Where's your Teddy, dolly, baby?
Bring it to Mommy.
Bring it here.
Come here.
Come to Mommy, Daddy.

Switch off the light . . . . on.
Shut the door.
Open the door.

Do you want to go out?
Do you want to go in the car?
Shall we go in the car?
Yes.   No.
Can you see the airplane?

Do you want to get up?
Do you want to get down?
Do you want to have a bath?

That's Mommy's.
It's hot. Ow!
Don't do that.

Stand up. Sit down.
Lie down. Sit up.
Give Mommy a kiss.

Hello. Hi.
Wave bye-bye.
Clap hands.
Play pat-a-cake.
Peep-boo. Peek-a-boo.

Here it is.
There it is.

Good girl, boy.
Bad girl, boy.

Hush, Baby's sleeping.
Wake up!
Go to sleep.
Put Teddy to sleep.

Do you want a drink (milk, juice)?
Do you want some dinner?
Do you want a banana?
Do you want some more?
Look, it's all gone.
You've finished it.

Look at the dog.
Look at it . . . . Look at that.

Put it back. Put it down.
No, don't touch.
Spit it out.
It's dirty (stones, sand).

What does the dog say!
. . . . woof.
What does the cat say?
. . . . meow.

Rhymes

Rock-a-bye baby.   Ride a cock-horse.   See-saw Margery Daw.

11. Language Development and Its Assessment

Regardless of their philosophical preference for one communication method over another, teachers of the hearing impaired would agree that their major concern is with language development. Some teachers have been prepared to trade speech for signs on the assumption that reading and writing skills would be markedly improved. Indeed, it is the prevailing low standards of reading and writing, accompanied by poor speech intelligibility, which have led to the recent massive swing away from oralism. Linguists, psychologists, and other newcomers to the field may be unaware that similar reasoning once led to the rejection of the "combined method" (oral plus manual) in favor of the "pure oral method." The re-introduction of sign language under the rubric "total communication" is a case of history repeating itself and is unlikely to lead to a general increase in reading achievement. Indeed, studies not yet published reveal that reading skills are more highly correlated with the use of speech than with signs.

Traditional Approaches to Language Teaching

The layman has difficulty in comprehending the nature and extent of the hearing-impaired person's problems. He may presume that vision can readily be substituted for audition. On the surface, it appears to be a question of communication which could be solved by the use of the written, rather than the spoken, word. Indeed, early attempts to educate deaf people relied almost entirely on writing, supplemented by spelling with a manual alphabet. Articulation was then taught on a letter-by-letter, or syllable-by-syllable basis. However, while it is relatively easy to teach a vocabulary of several hundred written or fingerspelled words when these words represent objects or actions, it is markedly more difficult to teach syntax, the rules by which sentences are constructed. How can one explain the use of words such as "the," "is," and "of"?

Two contrasting lines of attack have prevailed from the 17th century right through to the present day. These may be characterized as the grammatical, analytic, or structured approach versus the natural, global, conversational, or developmental approach. Each has had its protagonists, but rarely has either method been used to the exclusion of the other.

The Grammatical Method

The grammatical approach has involved the learning and classifying of words as nouns, verbs, prepositions and so on, then of learning their permitted positions in sentences as subject, verb, or object. Sometimes this has been done with the help of key question words such as Who, What, Where, and When (Fitzgerald, 1949), and sometimes by the memorization of basic sentence patterns. The terminology (or metalanguage) has changed over the years, in keeping with current usage. Hearing-impaired children of today may be familiar with terms such as noun phrase, verb phrase, kernel sentence, and perhaps even transformational grammar! The net result is often a young adult who can perform a wide range of grammatical operations, yet who is unable to construct reasonable sentences. Similar results are obtained with normal-hearing people exposed to a foreign language through a grammatical approach. When taught by this method, present tense can be converted to the future or the past; the active can be changed to the passive; a negative transformed to an interrogative; and yet conversation, even in simple phrases, is stilted and clumsy. In order to create a sentence, students taught by a grammatical approach engage mentally in the deliberate selection of parts of speech, tenses, and agreements. In spite of the major effort involved, their resulting utterances are often trivial or ill-formed, and communication is labored.

The Natural Method

Communicative need is generally the focus of concern for those using a so-called "natural" approach. The idea here is that language should be learned, rather than taught, much as the young normal-hearing child learns at his mother's knee. This method may be suitable when habilitation begins in a parent-infant program. However, problems abound when the child is no longer an infant or toddler, but a 4-, 5-, or 6-year-old child. Many of the relevant conditions for such a form of language learning are no longer "naturally" available and have to be contrived. The little child's bond with his mother provides a secure base from which he can experiment verbally with little fear of disapproval. A similar accepting attitude has to be present in the teacher, who in turn needs to be rewarded by the child's affection and respect.

The older child's motivation to learn language for communication purposes may be marginal if he has alternative means of satisfying his needs—either by acting independently or by communicating nonverbally. A further problem is that the "natural" method depends essentially on one-to-one communication such as occurs between parent and infant. How can one replicate this in the special classroom? It is rare indeed that all members of a class have identical interests and communicative needs. The abundant interaction which is possible (though not necessarily actual) between parent (as native speaker) and child is drastically reduced when the child becomes one of a class of non-users of the language with access to only one teacher and perhaps an assistant.

Historically, a "natural" approach has been used in conjunction with the written form, although the methods may appear incompatible. At a time when hearing aids were not available for children with profound hearing impairment, writing was used as an alternative to talking. This manner of teaching was possible when the child had a private tutor who interacted continuously by writing down everything that was happening. Language was taught through communication by the written word. A strong affective bond was forged between tutor and pupil, the tutor effectively becoming a companion or surrogate parent. Thus, the prerequisite conditions for language learning were essentially met.

A Guided Interactional Approach to Language Development

When habilitation of the hearing-impaired child and his family is begun in the first year or so of life, an approach to language learning that follows a normal developmental path is clearly appropriate. The parent, rather than the child, is seen as the target for training. With guidance such as described in the previous chapter, parents can be assisted to master techniques which will facilitate the optimal use of their child's sensory modalities, and the development of his motor-speech skills. Parents also need to learn how to interact with their child in a manner which will help him perceive the meaning of the language they use.

In guiding the development of spoken language in the young hearing-impaired child, several aspects have to be attended to concurrently. The child can be encouraged to listen and then look; to listen and then vocalize; or to listen and then show by his actions that he has understood what was said. Listening skills are developed in relation to babbling spontaneously at various times in the day; for the purpose of understanding what is said during most of the day; with reference to environmental sounds as they occur; and for music, singing, and dancing, according to desire. The actual sounds and language selected must be appropriate for the particular child in a given situation or at a specific time.

The crucial factors that determine whether a hearing-impaired child will acquire spoken language are the competence of the teacher/clinician and her ability to guide the parents, the extent to which the parents are able to understand and apply the principles of early language development, and the relative intactness of the child's brain and central nervous system.

A hearing-impaired child has reached the beginning stages of language learning when he looks at and/or listens to people when they talk, has a varied phonetic repertoire, communicates vocally, modifies his tone of voice to indicate his feelings, and gives evidence of symbolic behavior such as utilizing the conventional gestures of shaking his head to mean no, and nodding to mean yes. He is then ready to attach meanings to the sound patterns he and others make. Thus, the little child who is fond of going outdoors can be expected to learn to recognize the word "out" in the context "Do you want to go out?" through listening, speechreading, or both—if such a question has been asked each time his actions have indicated that this is what he would like to do.

Relating Language and Experience

Before a hearing-impaired child can be expected to understand particular words, phrases, or questions, he must have the opportunity to hear (or see) them literally hundreds of times in appropriate contexts (when these expressions are central to his needs and wants). The major differences between the normal-hearing and the hearing-impaired baby are that the former can hear over very much greater distances than the latter, and that the auditory pattern he receives is relatively clear and undistorted. The normal-hearing child is therefore more readily exposed to an abundance of spoken language and consequently is likely to learn more quickly than the hearing-impaired child. The parents of the hearing-impaired child therefore have to compensate for this problem by being almost constantly available and sufficiently close to the child so that he can hear, and if necessary see, the spoken patterns that refer clearly and simply to his focus of interest. Fortunately, the young child is curious about most aspects of the daily chores that mothers perform, so the essential repetition is ensured. This type of one-to-one interaction involves sensing the child's interest, telling him about it, and then waiting for his vocal commentary. It becomes quite tiring if one parent has to accept the entire responsibility.

Fathers, as well as mothers, should be encouraged to contribute on a daily basis. Once again, the strategy is to link language learning to routine activities. Shaving is such an activity. By rising 5 or 10 minutes earlier, father can put the hearing aids on the child and sit him nearby in his infant seat or high chair. While he shaves, father can talk to the child about what he is doing, put lather on the child's face, or let him hear and feel the noise of the electric shaver. He can let the child feel his face, rough beforehand and smooth afterwards. As the child becomes familiar with some of the vocabulary or phrases, new ones can be introduced.

Serious problems arise in providing adequate linguistic input if both parents work full-time. Sometimes the child's grandmother is available and willing to become a mother-substitute and to attend the guidance sessions. More often, a sitter or housekeeper is hired, often on a temporary basis. It is not easy to find a person who is willing to invest the necessary energy and devotion to the child's habilitation, over the two- to three-year period before the child is old enough to go to school. The problem is magnified if the person responsible for the child is not a native speaker of the language the child is to learn. Parents who wish their child to talk will soon see the wisdom of one of them being at home, if at all possible, during their child's preschool years.

Developing and Checking Language Comprehension

Like his normal-hearing counterpart, the hearing-impaired child at first relies on cues from the situation, the tone of voice with which he is addressed, the facial expression of the speaker, and any other visual information available. Such nonverbal cues are supplied liberally in the early months of habilitation. However, since it is our aim that the child learn to communicate verbally, his ability to understand spoken language without nonverbal cues must be checked periodically. Thus, in the beginning his mother asks, "Do you want a drink?" as she is offering him one. In this context, his comprehension is facilitated by seeing the bottle or cup. Later she must check his comprehension by asking the same question at a time when he is not anticipating a drink. Evidence of his comprehension could be the licking of his lips or looking toward the place where his drink usually comes from. Parents can be asked to write down the phrases they use most frequently in each of the routine situations such as washing, dressing, meal-times, and play, and enter the date when phrases are understood first with, and later without, nonverbal cues. Alternatively or additionally they can use a list such as is provided in the Appendix to the previous chapter. This procedure helps to alert parents to words and phrases which are commonly understood by young children but which may not be understood by their child.

Certain words and phrases are necessary for communication in the routine situations of the child's daily life, and teacher/clinicians should ensure that children in their care have sufficient exposure to them. The child should always be addressed by his name, so that he is quickly familiarized with it. He also needs to know the names of the important people in his environment, such as "Mommy," "Daddy," his brothers, sisters, and pets. Questions such as "Where's Daddy?" or "Where's Mommy?" should be asked frequently, with the answer "There he is" or "There she is" provided for him until he is able to respond without help. Similarly he can be asked to point out favorite toys or objects. These questions should not be asked simply in a test situation, where the objects are laid on a table or the people are sitting round the room. They should be built into natural situations or games such as "Hide and Seek." The little child enjoys running to find the person or object requested. As the child's vocabulary of names and objects increases, he should be helped to respond to the questions "What's that?," "Who's that?," and "What is . . . doing?" By helping the child understand and respond appropriately to questions, he will be led to ask them in order to obtain information for himself. Examples of questions and answers are provided in Table 11.A.

The teacher/clinician also needs to monitor the type of semantic notions which the child is developing. Is his comprehension limited to names of people and objects, or does he also understand the meaning of words such as "no," "more," "all-gone," "up," "on," "off," "out," and "hot" when they occur in phrases or sentences? During the guidance session, the teacher/clinician can demonstrate ways in which parents can check their child's comprehension and can determine the extent to which the child needs to supplement auditory patterns with speechreading.

TABLE 11.A
First Questions and Some Answers

Questions	Answers
Where's (Daddy)?	There. Over there.
Where's the . . . ?	All gone. Upstairs.
What's that?	Name of object.
Is it a . . . ?	Yes. No.
Who's that?	Name of person.
Is it (Barbara)?	Yes. No.
Do you want (some more)?	Yes. No. Some, no more.
Do you want a/the/some . . . ?	Yes. No.
Do you want this one?	Yes. No. This one.
Do you want to (go out)?	Yes. No. (Go out).
Do you want Mummy to (open it)?	Yes. No. (Open it).
Do you want this one or that one?	This one. That one.
Do you want a . . . or a . . . ?	Name of object.
What do you want?	Name of food, toy, etc.

Developing and Checking the Child's Use of Language

We encourage parents to write down each word, phrase, or approximation as it becomes stabilized in their child's vocabulary.

Single words such as those mentioned above are commonly among those spoken by a normal-hearing child. They are also important for a hearing-impaired child and he should be helped to use them in the course of everyday activities. By questioning, the teacher/clinician can find out what sounds are entering the child's phonology. Does he say / ɔ / for "off," /baba/ for "mama," and /o/ or /no/ for "no"? At this point, the teacher/clinician has the opportunity to encourage transfer of sounds from the child's phonetic to his phonologic repertoire. The more accurate the child's pronunciation of words becomes, the easier it will be for others to understand what he says. It will also help him to retrieve a word from long-term memory when he wants to compare it with a new, somewhat similar word. Should a sound such as [f] not be present in the phonetic repertoire of the child who is approximating the word "off," the teacher/clinician will be spurred to develop it phonetically and transfer it into the child's phonology as quickly as possible. Parents are thus encouraged to listen carefully to what their children say. A few choose to learn the phonetic alphabet used in this book.

Teacher/clinicians and parents should not be surprised if the hearing-impaired child uses only vowels or single syllables in his early approximations, if the phonetic nature of the approximation changes from one week to another, or even if words which were commonly used for a few weeks disappear from his expressive vocabulary. Normal-hearing children pass through a similar phase of development. Parents and teachers of hearing-impaired children tend to become anxious and may react by putting pressure on their children to name objects repeatedly, or to imitate words in which they are no longer interested. Such a procedure runs the risk of stopping the free flow of the child's communication.

By the time the child has a vocabulary of about 50 words, it becomes helpful to check them from a list of 500 words and, as his vocabulary continues to increase, to use a 2,000-word list (Ling & Ling, 1977). Parents record whether a word is understood with or without cue and whether it is imitated or used spontaneously. The teacher/clinician goes over the list with the parent and confirms for herself any words which she feels may be understood only with cue. The point of this type of assessment is not to give an absolutely accurate count of the child's vocabulary, but rather to determine whether it is growing at an adequate rate and whether there are any obvious gaps which require special attention. Does the child use verbs, adjectives, negatives, question words, function words, and demonstratives, as well as nouns? Does he use verbs such as *want, need, get, like,* and *have* in addition to verbs like *run, jump,* and *walk?* Our language thesaurus lists words by topic, according to their frequency of usage by young normal-hearing children, and provides examples of phrases in which the words have somewhat different meanings. It is especially useful to those whose native language is not English.

Word combinations may be expected to be spoken by a hearing-impaired child only after he has developed a sizeable vocabulary of single words which he uses freely in interacting with friends and family. The teacher/clinician can point out to parents that the normal-hearing child may have as many as 250 words in his expressive vocabulary before he attempts to formulate phrases. For both the normal-hearing and the hearing-impaired child, the earliest form of two-word combinations is a simple listing of words, such as "Daddy shoe," and it is only in observing the situation that the child's intention can be inferred. Thus he may be pointing out Daddy's shoe or asking Daddy to help him take his shoe off. The child's behavior indicates an awareness of the relationship between the objects, but he is unable to express it linguistically. To do this he has to have a 2-year-old level of cognitive maturity. In addition, articulatory skill is required to indicate the possessive, as in "Daddy's." Function words, however, are of major importance in the expression of semantic relations. Only when the child's single-word vocabulary includes function words will he be in a position to combine them with content words. He cannot be expected to say "more juice" if he has never said "more," or to say "sock off" if he has never used the word "off."

The teacher/clinician may have to intervene in order to ensure that the hearing-impaired child does not remain at the single-word stage for an unduly long period. She can demonstrate that by changing stress and intonation patterns, function words can be drawn to the child's attention. The natural tendency is to stress content, rather than function, words in a sentence, e.g., "Take your *shoes* off," "Put your *coat* on," or "Put it in the *box*." However, it is easy to change the focus and say, "Can you take your shoes *off*? That's right. Take them *off*. *Off* they come." "Put your coat *on*. Put it *on*." "Put it *in* the box. *In* it goes." One can almost sing the crucial words in order to give them salience.

Provided with many such models as part of the daily routine, the hearing-impaired child is likely to produce some phrases himself. As he tugs and pulls to get his overboots off, he is likely to call for help, approximating either one word or another. If he says "boot," his mother can respond by saying "Yes, that's your boot," without moving to help him. He may then say "off," in which case she can say "Oh, you want Mummy to take your boot off," and perhaps she can elicit *"boot off"* as she helps him off with it. While the child is young, he needs help in dressing and undressing, and so there are hundreds of opportunities for him to learn the appropriate language. Once he becomes independent, as we wish him to, such language would have to be taught in contrived situations.

Just as the young normal-hearing child is not constantly corrected for faults of articulation or syntax, neither should the hearing-impaired child be. Errors should be accepted as part of the learning process. The rewards of communicating easily in the language spoken by his family and by his peers are usually sufficient to spur the child. Correction of errors of fact are in order, as when the child uses the word "dog" in reference to a wolf. An appropriate response would be "It looks like a dog, but we call it a *wolf.*"

Deliberate attempts by parents to teach elaborate polite question forms, such as "May I have a cookie, please?" are likely to lead to failure or frustration for hearing-impaired children who are only at a single-word or two-word level. An acceptable utterance would be "want cookie" or "cookie, please." They are quite unable to handle the length or complexity of the complete question form either in terms of its language structure or the coordinated articulation it requires.

The skillful use of questions by teacher/clinicians and parents can assist the child to advance to the use of kernel sentences. Kernel sentences, while they may not be grammatically correct, contain the basic constituents of a sentence, namely a subject and a predicate. In response to the child's "go work," his mother may try to elicit the subject of the sentence by saying, "Who's going to work?" If the child says "Daddy," his mother can then reply, "Yes, Daddy's going to work." The child may then say "Daddy go work," producing a kernel sentence. If the child says "doggie eating" as he watches a dog eating his bone, his mother can say, "The dog's eating what?" and may elicit "eating bone." She can then say, "You tell Daddy . . . The doggie's eating a bone." The child may thus be encouraged to produce a kernel sentence—subject, verb, object—"doggie eat bone."

Situations in which the child is highly motivated to communicate should be exploited to the utmost. The highest level of spoken language capabilities can usually be insisted on. Thus, in his great desire to get outdoors, the child may be rather easily led into using whatever words and phrases he has at his disposal. If he stands by the door saying "go out," his mother may say, *"Who* wants to go out? You want *Daddy* to go out? You want *Mommy* to go out?"* Because he is eager to go, he may well figure out an expanded form and say *"me* go out" or *"Bobby* go out," and be rewarded by being permitted to go out to play. This strategy is more likely to lead the child to think about what he needs to say in order to communicate his ideas. If his mother were to tell him, "Say, I want to go out" and expect him to imitate it, he may simply be unable to do so because both the length and the complexity of the sentence are beyond him. The over-use of imitation as a strategy for developing the child's language may create problems in that the purpose of spoken language—communication—is forgotten. On the other hand, imitation is helpful in developing motor speech patterns.

Special language training programs, many of which involve imitation, have been devised for children with serious language delay, but normal hearing. Such children might be emotionally disturbed, cognitively impaired, autistic, brain-damaged, environmentally deprived, or may have no other symptoms than the language delay itself. Recent advances in psycholinguistics have led to changes in the content of their language training. Rather than emphasize the teaching of syntactic structures in the early stages, the focus is upon the expression of semantic relationships. Rather than attempt to teach complete sentences such as "This is a ball," "I have a car," or "The boy is running," the teacher/clinician or parent provides the child with reduced models to imitate. These models exemplify semantic relations such as possession ("Mommy book"), actor-action (boy run) or location (in car) and may not be given in correct English. For children with limited cognitive and linguistic potential, such an approach may be justified. However, the use of such a technique with hearing-impaired children would seem unwise. First, the normal-hearing child with serious language delay would usually have access to normal patterns of spoken language outside the training session, whereas the hearing-impaired child, because of his limited hearing, does not. Second, the focus is on production, with little attention being paid to comprehension. Third, the adult's presentation of reduced forms in language training in an imitation paradigm seems unlikely to result in the child's becoming able to formulate his own well-formed sentences. Fourth, given the hearing-impaired child's tendency to retain rather rigidly what he has been taught, it would seem to be a poor strategy to deliberately teach him to imitate and produce incorrect forms which he later has to unlearn. This point of view should not be taken to mean that nothing less than complete sentences should be accepted from the hearing-impaired child, but rather that he should be exposed to normal models.

Assessing Spoken Syntax

As soon as the hearing-impaired child is talking abundantly, it becomes worthwhile to undertake a formal analysis of a sample of his spoken language. The purpose of such an analysis is to assess the child's status at the beginning of a teaching year, select syntactic structures which should be emerging in the child's language, and evaluate his performance after a period of training. This type of analysis could also be used for research purposes, such as comparing progress made by children taught by different methods (for example, structured versus unstructured teaching).

Several standard techniques which have been developed for use with children who have severe language disorders are also suitable for use with hearing-impaired children. One such approach (Lee, 1974) will be discussed in this chapter. Others will be listed in the bibliography together with sources of information about alternative tests and procedures. The major disadvantage of assessing language by means of analyzing a spoken language sample is the amount of time involved, which is usually about three to four hours. This is counteracted by the precision with which one can determine suitable language goals. Furthermore, this technique can be used repeatedly without the child becoming bored. Few standardized tests are appropriate for hearing-impaired children, and repeated use may produce invalid results.

Lee proposes two forms of Developmental Sentence Analysis: Developmental Sentence Types and Developmental Sentence Scoring. *Developmental Sentence Types* permits a child's pre-sentence utterances to be classified and entered on a chart at one of three levels: single words, two-word combinations, and constructions which do not contain a noun (or pronoun) and verb in a subject-predicate relationship. Each level is subdivided to enable the teacher/clinician to record an utterance as one of five types. At the single-word level, these are noun, designator (here, there, this, that), descriptive item, verb, and vocabulary item. Elaborations of these basic forms are specified for two-word combinations, and constructions.

Developmental Sentence Scoring was devised for evaluating the grammatical structure of the language of children who talk in "complete" sentences. Lee uses the word "complete" to describe a sentence having a subject and predicate even though it may not be grammatically correct. Sentences in the language sample are examined with respect to the presence of the following eight categories: indefinite pronouns or noun modifiers, personal pronouns, main verbs, secondary verbs, negatives, conjunctions, interrogative reversals, and wh- questions. A score (from 1 to 8) is provided for each of a variety of grammatical forms under each category. Thus the pronouns *I, me, my, mine, you, and your(s)* are given a score of 1 because they are used by very young children, whereas *(his) own, one, oneself, whichever, whoever,* and *whatever* occur much later and consequently are assigned a weighting of 7. Lee provides a chart which shows the position of various grammatical forms in the developmental progression. A score of 1 is added to each sentence which is correct in every respect. This procedure is used to account for structures such as articles and prepositions which do not appear as a category. A sentence score is calculated and can be compared with normative data obtained from 200 children aged 2 years 0 months to 6 years 11 months.

A tape-recorded sample of 100 utterances is recommended for using the Developmental Sentence Types protocol, whereas 50 are considered sufficient to obtain a valid assessment with the Developmental Sentence Scoring method. For either type of analysis, the sample should be collected during a single session of one hour, consisting of informal play and conversation. The teacher/clinician is encouraged to elicit the highest level of language of which the child is capable. The utterances to be analyzed should be consecutive. Repetitions and imitations are excluded, however, as are recitations.

The person who collects the language sample transcribes it into English orthography (spelling). Because the purpose of the analysis is to study the child's syntax, rather than his articulation, a phonetic transcription is not recommended. However, careful listening is essential if the child is not to be credited with grammatical forms he does not yet possess, e.g., plurals and verb tenses. Teacher/clinicians who are using the phonologic evaluation recommended in Chapter 9 of this book could utilize one language sample for both a phonologic and linguistic analysis.

How often should a language sample be subjected to the in-depth type of analysis proposed by Lee? She suggests once every three months for children with language disorders. Because the transcription of hearing-impaired children's speech is so time consuming, even when English orthography is used, a twice yearly analysis might be considered adequate, with a shortened version used during the intervening periods. It makes little sense to invest several hours on analysis and planning if this time has to be spread over several weeks. Children with moderate to severe hearing impairment may make more rapid progress than the analyst!

Developing Syntactic Structures

The particular value of Lee's system is that the teacher/clinician can locate on the chart those structures the child uses accurately; those which are attempted; and those which occur next in the developmental progression for each of the categories, and which should be the targets for subsequent development. Thus it might be noted that although the child is using the root form of many verbs such as "fall," "go," "run," and "break," he does not use the copula "is."

The normal-hearing child uses the copula "is," as in "It is big," or "It's heavy," and the auxiliary "is" as in "The boy is running" in his early sentences. Unfortunately, the word "is" is usually un-stressed; in addition, it has mainly high-frequency components and may only be audible to a hearing-impaired child if it is spoken close to the microphone of his hearing aid. If he has no hearing for the upper frequencies, it may be completely inaudible. Fur-thermore, the word "is" is difficult to speechread. Most hearing-impaired children will therefore require some assistance in estab-lishing it in their phonology.

The first step would seem to be to develop [ɪz] phonetically. Word-final /s/ and /z/ are very important in English phonology since they are used to mark plurals, possessives, and verb forms, in addition to being present in words such as "Yes." The hearing-impaired child who can babble these sounds and produce them automatically will be aided enormously in acquiring good spoken English. Only when the child can produce [ɪz] phonetically, should his attention be drawn to it linguistically. Slight stress on the word may help. "That *is* hot." Greater salience is achieved by using it as the first word in an utterance, as in the question forms "*Is* it a car?", "*Is* it a dog?", "*Is* it hot?", "*Is* it blue?" The questions can be asked as part of a game in which the child hides an object in a bag and his mother attempts to guess what it is. The child can at first respond "Yes" or "No," or maybe "Yes . . . car," "No(t) dog." The child can then take his turn at guessing what his mother has hidden. She can use the longer responses "Yes it *is*," or "It is not." Later she might vary her wording to "It's a _____," "No, it's not," or "No, it isn't."

Analysis of a spoken language sample may reveal that few pronouns are used. This is not surprising when one considers that such words as *he, she, it, we, they,* etc. contain principally high-frequency components, are of brief duration, and are frequently unstressed. A poorly developed pronoun system remains typical of the special school pupil, even of high-school age. This may be because pronouns have been taught through written exercises in which the child is asked to replace nouns in a given sentence. The hearing-impaired child often completes such exercises in a mechanical way, without involving his thought processes.

The manner in which normal-hearing children learn to utilize pronouns is very different. When talking to toddlers, parents tend to avoid pronouns, presumably in an effort to facilitate comprehension. Thus a mother will refer to herself by name, as in "*Mommy's* going out now," instead of saying "*I'm* going . . . ," "That's *Mommy's* book" rather than "That's *my* book." Similarly she will use the child's name when addressing him, "That's *Peter's* book," rather than "That's *your* book." She may even point to herself or the child to prevent any ambiguity. Sometimes the young child's mother provides both forms as models, one immediately following the other, as in "That's Mommy's. It's *mine*.", "This is Peter's. It's *yours*." The young normal-hearing child first uses his own name to identify himself, as in "John do it." He may additionally say "Me do it" and only later will he begin to produce "I" when referring to himself. He continues to use his own name in this way until he is about 3 years old.

The hearing-impaired child should be permitted to follow the normal stages of development, so that he begins to construct his own phrases, those he understands, such as "Brian play ball." It is harmful to insist that a child at this stage should repeat a correct sentence such as "I am playing ball" which includes not only the unfamiliar pronoun "I" but also the auxiliary "am" plus the main verb with its obligatory ending, -*ing*, neither of which he has mastered. Furthermore, when the parent or teacher/clinician says to the child, "Say, I am playing ball," the child may reasonably become confused, since the "I" no longer refers to him!

The pronouns "he" and "she" can be developed as responses to questions such as "Who has . . . ?" (see Table 11.B for sample questions and answers). The game "Picture Lotto," which can be

TABLE 11.B
Question Forms for Eliciting Pronouns

Questions	Answers
Who has the . . . ?	I have. You have. He/she has.
Who wants more? Who wants a (candy)? Who likes . . . ?	I do. He/she does.
Who did that? Who (broke) the . . . ? Who (spilled) the . . . ?	I did. You did. He/she did. Not me. Not you.
Does (Daddy) like . . . ? Does (Mommy) like . . . ? Does (Robert) want . . . ? Does (Mary) need . . . ?	Yes, he does. Yes, she does. No, he doesn't. No, she doesn't.
Who can . . . ? Can (John) (run)? Can (Jane) (swim)?	I/you/he/she can. Yes, he can. No, he can't. Yes, she can. No, she can't.

enjoyed from age 3, can be adapted to develop the accurate use of pronouns. Three or four players are required, at least one male and one female, to allow for reference to *I, you, he,* and *she.* Each player has a card with several pictures on it. Separate matching pictures are placed in a bag. One player selects a card from the bag and, without showing it to the others, asks "Who has the . . . ?" or "Who's got the . . . ?" The person who has the matching picture on his card, let's say it is Daddy, calls out, "I have." The child's mother can then say "*I* haven't got it. *You* haven't got it. *He* has it" (pointing to Daddy). In this manner, the child can have lots of exposure to the new pronouns in the context "he has" and "she has" which contrast with the forms "I have" and "you have," which the child already uses. With practice occurring naturally as part of the game, the child himself will begin to use the pronouns. The alert parent can give the new pronouns extra stress when they are appropriate in other situations and try to elicit them from the child.

Variations of the Picture Lotto game permit the players only to listen, or to listen and speechread. The language patterns can be chosen to suit the hearing-impaired child's current capabilities. Played as suggested, Picture Lotto involves the hearing-impaired child in active listening, understanding, thinking, and speaking. He is exposed to sentence patterns which are transformed from question to statement, from positive to negative, and in which first one pronoun is used, then another.

The pronouns "he" and "she" can also be developed through the question form "Does . . . like?" Using a picture book containing pictures of foods and drinks, the child's mother can begin by checking that he can respond appropriately to the question "Do *you* like . . . ?" with "I do" or "I don't," as well as with "Yes" and "No." His mother can point to each picture in turn and ask "Do *you* like . . . ?" The child is then encouraged to take his turn at asking. The form "You like . . . ?" may be accepted at this stage. Mother and child can then compare their respective likes and dislikes and then proceed to discuss those of other family members, one at a time. The interaction might continue as follows:

Mother: What about Daddy? Does Daddy like this [pointing to picture]?

Child: Yes.

Mother: *He* does! Daddy likes it.
Does Daddy like that [pointing to a different picture]?

Child: I don't know.

Mother: Go ask Daddy. Show him all the pictures.
(Child goes to find Daddy)

Child: Daddy, you like this?

Daddy: Mmm, yeah, I like it.

Child: You like that?

Daddy: Ugh, no, I don't.

etc.

(Child returns to Mother)

Mother: Well, did you find out? Let's see. Does Daddy like this?
Child: Yes.
Mother: *He* does! Does Daddy like this?
Child: Yes.
Mother: *He* does. Does *he* like that?
Child: No.
Mother: *He* doesn't. *I* do. Do *you*?
Child: I like it.
Mother: Let's see all the things that Daddy likes. *He* likes this. *He* likes that. Now you tell me some more.

The child is then encouraged to try. Note that the names of the foods were not used in this particular conversation. This technique helps to focus on the structures being developed without any interference from vocabulary items with which the child may be unfamiliar or be unable to pronounce. Conversational work on the question forms "Do you like?" and "Does he like?" could be complemented by reading to the child the nonsense story by Dr. Seuss entitled "Green Eggs and Ham." Hearing-impaired children find it hilarious to ask or to be asked, "Do you like green eggs and ham?"

Pronouns should only be used when their reference has been made quite clear to the child. Similarly, if he uses a pronoun without identifying his reference, he should be asked to do so. Thus, if the child who has been playing with several friends comes to his mother howling "He push(ed) me," he should be asked "*Who* pushed you?" On being told "Robert," his mother's response might then be, "Oh, *Robert* pushed you. *He* is rough. Did *he* hurt you? *He* is a bad boy." Appropriate dialogues can be worked out to highlight whatever new structure is, or should be, emerging in the child's language.

In this section we have given but a few examples of how syntactic structures might be developed. The parent or inexperienced teacher/clinician will necessarily find this information incomplete. However, a more in-depth presentation would require a book, backed up by further research. We would like to emphasize that guided language work will be most effective when planned and carried out on an individual basis, or with groups of two or three children having similar needs. In Chapter 13 we discuss how certain types of educational settings facilitate or prevent this type of teaching. In any event, parents should be maximally involved in their children's language programs from infancy to adulthood.

Issues Relating to Language Development for Late Starters

A severely hearing-impaired child whose family has not received guidance before the child's third birthday can be considered a late starter, as by age 3 the normal-hearing child is already talking in sentences. The late starter is at risk of going through life with a permanent, severe language deficiency. Clearly, if the child is 5 or 6 years old, the case is more serious. It is, of course, possible to develop good spoken language even with such a late start, but intensive work is required by a highly competent teacher, preferably with the parents playing a strongly supportive role. The question is how best to do it. Is a guided interactional approach, based on normal spoken language development, feasible, or should formal instruction, emphasizing the written form, be employed? A brief review of several related topics follows.

Techniques of Foreign Language Teaching

Techniques utilized in the teaching of foreign languages to normal-hearing people have had considerable influence on the practices of teachers of the hearing impaired. The grammatical approach has a very long history, continuing to the present day. Foreign languages are more often taught to adults and adolescents than to young children, and so a formal, grammatical or analytical approach may be considered both efficient and appropriate. The adult's greater cognitive abilities can be harnessed to the task. Often the aim is to teach the student to read and write the foreign language, rather than to speak it. Generally, the student is first taught the alphabet and phonetic repertoire of the new language, usually with reference to his native language. Vocabulary lists are committed to memory, each word in the new language being paired to one in the old. Words may include numbers, colors, days of the week, the months and seasons, and common objects in the home and classroom. A number of stock phrases such as those commonly used in greeting and leave-taking are taught. Rote memory (the declension of nouns and conjugation of verbs) plays a large role. Translation to and from the new and native language is practiced. While the normal-hearing person might develop fair competence in reading and writing the foreign language after five or six years of study, he rarely becomes able to converse fluently. The average hearing-impaired child, however, without a native spoken language as a base for comparison, is barely literate even after as many as 12 years of formal schooling.

With the advent of mass international travel, an audiolingual approach to foreign language teaching has become common. As its title suggests, the emphasis is on listening and talking. Using programmed tape-recordings or disks, the student initially learns to imitate the sounds of the new language (with or without reference to the written form). Soon he is introduced to phrases, often in the context of brief conversations. The student listens and repeats, over and over again. Basic sentence patterns are taught by rote. Model questions and answers are provided. The student listens to both, then to the question only. He gives his own response and compares it with the model answer. Sentence patterns of increasing complexity are gradually introduced. Although it is possible for students to progress at their own rate through the program, individual needs and interests are not accounted for, since it is a preplanned program.

Unfortunately, the introduction of the audiolingual approach has not led to large numbers of people becoming fluent users of the foreign language they studied. The ability to speak in a controlled context under the teacher's guidance does not seem to generalize to greater freedom of expression any more readily than does the grammar-translation approach. The emphasis on rote memory and mimicry probably acts counter to the development of conversational fluency. While native speakers in real-life situations have many possible options in the wording they use to ask or answer a question, the typical language program tends to offer only a few stereotyped patterns. Hearing-impaired children may also be taught to memorize basic sentence patterns through the written form, rather than through hearing. Their responses are written, rather than spoken. The children become proficient at forming their own sentences based on the given models. Once again, however, difficulty is encountered in communication.

Teachers of foreign languages have identified some of the reasons why relatively few people learn a second language in a classroom situation. First of all, the classroom does not provide the type of social interaction in which language learning is likely to flourish. In the event that the class consists entirely of novices, the teacher, the "authority figure," may be forced into doing most of the talking, and learning from peers is thus precluded. In the typical class, there is often little motivation to learn. Both adolescents and adults usually feel uncomfortable about attempting to speak a language when they have not mastered the sound system and cannot construct sensible sentences. The teacher's function is usually thought to include the presentation of graduated lessons in pronunciation, vocabulary, and grammar, and subsequently to correct her students' faulty attempts at speaking and writing. Knowing that they are almost certain to make errors of one sort or other, students tend to be inhibited about talking in the new language. Much of the class time is expended with students taking turns haltingly translating or producing sentences, while the others wait and, supposedly, listen. The student has greater exposure to poor than to good models, and peer-to-peer communication is inevitably in the first language. The situation in special classes for hearing-impaired children has often much in common with the "sure fail" tactics of the type of foreign language teaching described above.

Immersion courses are another form of foreign language teaching. The use of the word "immersion" is misleading: Although all teaching is undertaken in the target language, none of the students is a native speaker of the language to be learned; only the teacher is. Hearing-impaired children attending special schools or classes are in essentially the same kind of situation. Here, too, there is only one native speaker, the teacher, and again there are no peer models. The teacher has to carry the enormous responsibility of providing all of the language input. The teacher is active and the children, although they may imitate, are essentially passive. Communication between hearing-impaired children in beginning classes is inevitably nonverbal. Unless parents, teacher aides, or normal-talking children spend considerable time in the special classroom, the hearing-impaired child is rarely in a position to witness or overhear examples of the varied types of verbal interchange which normally take place between native speakers of the language. Like his hearing counterpart in most foreign language courses, the hearing-impaired child is not in a position to pick up colloquial chit-chat, slang, or swearing, since these would not be considered appropriate for classroom teaching.

Foreign languages can be learned without formal instruction. The ideal situation is probably when the individual goes to live with a family in a community where only the new language is spoken. Student exchange programs, where an English child, for instance, goes to live with a French family, attempt this approach, but the duration of stay is generally far too brief; to have any effect, a minimum of three or four months would be required. Other possibilities include going to school or joining an activity group where most others in the setting speak the target language. In such situations, most of the prerequisite conditions for spoken language development are met: the language is learned in a social context; there is abundant interaction with native speakers, often on a one-to-one basis; the target language is the only major mode of communication; there is opportunity to learn casually from peers; communicative needs occur frequently and the motivation to acquire competence is high; the focus is on daily living and shared pleasures, not on language as a subject for study. A comparable situation occurs when a hearing-impaired child lives at home with his family and attends a regular nursery or kindergarten. However, because of his sensory deficit, support and guidance from a highly skilled teacher/clinician are required for the child, his family, and his other teachers to ensure their understanding of the nature and implications of his problem. They need to be informed about how they can assist the child in making optimal use of his perceptual capacities, and to be alerted to conversational strategies which should facilitate the child's acquisition of spoken language.

Teachers of second languages are now studying the manner in which first languages are acquired. They have become increasingly aware that languages have to be learned, rather than taught; that the rules have to be derived, rather than provided; and that the typical classroom lacks many of the prerequisite conditions for such learning to occur. One response has been to attempt to engineer communication situations (or transactions) which simulate those in which the language learner wishes to become competent. This "transactional engineering" approach emphasizes that there is much more involved than acquiring the phonology, semantics, and syntax of the language. The novice has also to discover pragmatic and socio-linguistic aspects of communication, i.e., how and when certain sentence patterns and expressions are used and how native speakers interact with one another in a variety of situations. We will come back to this topic later, with reference to hearing-impaired children.

Babbling and Language Development

In the event that training is not begun until the child is 3 or 4 years old, and even more so if he is already 5 or 6, neither teacher nor parent may feel that it is either possible or worthwhile to attempt to retrace the usual developmental steps in acquiring the prerequisite auditory-vocal skills. The direct teaching of language is immediately undertaken. We consider this to be a mistake.

The period of apprenticeship through babbling and vocal play is usually denied such children because babbling is considered to be babyish and demeaning. The child himself is not likely to conceive of babbling as infantile, but will quickly come to believe it to be so if important adults (parents or teachers) or older children tease or ridicule him when he babbles or jargons. Perhaps the older child's teachers or parents fear that babbling beyond the infant stage is an indicator of mental retardation and that silence is less embarrassing. However, as with other skills involving muscular co-ordination (playing the piano, ballet dancing, athletics, etc.), high levels of proficiency cannot be achieved without practicing scales or exercises.

Babbling may, in fact, be used by normal-hearing children well beyond the first year of life. It offers a means of experimenting with phonetic and phonologic aspects not only of their native language, but also in the learning of foreign language. Our son Philip, for example, has explored several languages through babble: his native language English, French at age 6, Russian at age 14, and most recently, German at age 17. It would be interesting to know if self-directed babbling accelerates language learning. Certainly the integration of auditory and articulatory patterns would appear to be facilitated by such practice.

Babbling can even be acceptable behavior for an adult. The mimicry of dialects and accents is somewhat similar to babbling and is a useful asset for teachers of speech. In reproducing another's faulty speech pattern, one may gain insight into how it was articulated and therefore be more able to devise appropriate remedial strategies. An example of public acceptance of babble is the popularity of a group of vocalists who sing Bach fugues to "doobeedoobeedoo . . ." The singing of newly learned babble patterns could also be enjoyed by older hearing-impaired children. An explanation of the rationale behind babble practice could lead to its acceptance by teen-agers and young adults who are seriously motivated to improve their articulation.

Extended babble practice guided by the teacher/clinician should permit a young hearing-impaired child to develop control over his articulatory muscles. During such practice the child is freed from the need to think about the linguistic structure of what he is saying. The practice of trying to correct both speech and language during communication is disastrous. Children who are subject to such treatment may be expected to reject verbal communication.

Bilingualism

Normal children exposed to a single language can usually master the basic skills in the first three years of life. It may take them about five years to master two languages when both are used from birth. Children with less than normal intellectual ability and those who have speech, hearing, or learning disorders, are likely to fail to master either language when exposed to both from infancy.

The outlook for a profoundly hearing-impaired child who receives his education in a language different from that used in his home is very poor. It is not just a difference of language, but also a difference of culture. Parents of foreign language background may be alienated if they are told that they must stop using that language at home and use only the language in which the hearing-impaired child is to be educated. Many are unable to follow this dictum because they cannot speak the new language; others may feel that they would be rejected by their own linguistic community.

When the hearing impairment is diagnosed, parents of foreign language background require careful counseling, with the help of an interpreter, if necessary. It is crucial that they gain a reasonable understanding of the extent of the impairment and the implications for the acquisition of spoken language and future education.

The child about 3 years of age who is diagnosed as having a moderate loss will probably have acquired some of the basic skills of his native language. It would probably be most beneficial to enroll him in a program which concentrated initially on providing guidance to the parents. An immediate aim would be promoting the development of the *native* language, together with establishing good psycho-social adjustment in the child and his parents. Prior to entry to kindergarten, the child should be introduced to the new language through individual tutoring in a play situation, and through attendance at a nursery school where he can learn from normal-speaking peers.

For the child who has not developed any spoken language by the time hearing impairment is diagnosed, the situation is very different. Such a child would likely have a severe to profound impairment, making mastery of language an arduous, long-term proposition even when learning conditions are otherwise ideal. Given that regular entry to school is at age 5, there is not the remotest possibility that a profoundly hearing-impaired child could match the normal-hearing child and master two languages. Rather than start teaching the family language, it makes more sense to help parents to realize that the child will require all available time and energy to learn the language in which he is scheduled to receive schooling. Once basic mastery of that language has been achieved, the family language can reasonably be introduced. When the hearing impairment is diagnosed in the first year or so of life, the parents would conceivably have time to learn the new language and keep ahead of their baby's needs. Providing parental attitude is favorable, ways and means can be found to ensure that the hearing-impaired child has access to a sufficiency of the desired language.

Sign Language

In families where both parents are deaf, and where sign language is their major means of communication, the situation for the normal-hearing child is to some extent comparable to the child who learns one language at home and then has to learn a new language at school. Deaf parents, however, will usually do their best to ensure that the hearing child learns to talk in very early childhood, since he then becomes especially valuable as an intermediary or interpreter. Hearing-impaired children will easily learn sign language from their parents, but if hearing aids and spoken language are not introduced until the child is 3 or 4 years old, he will have missed the optimal years for developing hearing and speech skills.

It has been claimed that spoken language can be taught more readily to hearing-impaired children who are already familiar with sign language. Spoken language is then viewed as a foreign language and sign language as the native language. However, sign language and spoken language are much more different than, say, English and Chinese. Sign language depends on vision and utilizes conventionalized gestures in space. Spoken languages normally depend on audition and involve arbitrary uses of pitch and loudness over time. The temporal order, or sequence, of the spoken sounds is crucial to their meaning. Sign language has its own syntax and its own semantic fields, neither of which correspond with spoken languages. Sign language has no phonology.

The child who uses sign language will be oriented to a system of coding and memorizing which is not compatible with that required for verbal learning involving either written or spoken language. The hearing-impaired child who is a native user of sign language will tend to filter the spoken or written language through his first language. Further, a hearing-impaired child who signs is unlikely to be readily motivated to switch to the much more complicated system of spoken language for which he receives only partial information. The deliberate initial use of sign language is not recommended, except where this is the family language.

Programmed Instruction

During the 1960s, programmed instruction emerged as a promising educational tool, and it was only natural that it should be applied in teaching language to hearing-impaired children. It has been successfully used in the teaching of a vocabulary of nouns, verbs, and adjectives through picture-word associations. Simple sentence structures have also been taught. Basically, programmed instruction follows a grammatical approach to language teaching, with its inherent problems. It seems designed to perpetuate—rather than remediate or prevent—some of the undesirable characteristics of "deaf" language, such as the use of stereotyped sentences. Common faults such as the indiscriminate use of the determiners "a" and "the," and the inappropriate reference of personal and relative pronouns, cannot be dealt with in single sentences. Only the larger context of a paragraph or conversation will determine whether "a" or "the" is correct. Such pragmatic aspects of language can best be learned through communication.

Pragmatic and Socio-linguistic Aspects of Communication

Proficiency in spoken language includes being able to carry on a two-way conversation: *understanding* what others say (this involves being able to perceive by hearing and/or speechreading); *speaking* clearly enough for others to understand (this involves mastery of the phonology, semantics, and syntax of the language plus the necessary articulatory skills); *comprehending* conversational topics appropriate to one's age and culture; *knowing* the ways in which conversations are entered upon, how new subjects are introduced, how conversations are concluded and leave-takings made; how information can be sought; how clarification can be obtained; how strangers or older people as distinct from friends or peers should be addressed. The so-called social graces depend largely on verbal skills, skills which the hearing-impaired child requires if he is to be readily accepted by his peers and elders.

Thought, Memory, and Language

The relationship between thought and language has been the subject of considerable controversy. It has been argued that higher levels of thought are not possible without language, and alternatively that the development of language depends on cognitive capacities. Parents and teachers of hearing-impaired children have long known intuitively that the most highly intelligent are not always those with the best language. Practical reasoning can be largely nonverbal in nature. While acknowledging the importance of nonverbal thinking, which is often artistic, creative, practical or mechanical, we plead that the hearing-impaired child be given the opportunity to develop verbal skills sufficient to give him access to science, medicine, literature, and culture.

Different perceptual and cognitive strategies are brought into action by the hearing-impaired language learner according to the type of input (written, signed, spoken, etc.) he receives, and upon his sensory capacities. Failure to stimulate the auditory system in infancy may limit the child to the use of visually based codes which tend to be iconic and spatial, well-suited to the recall of faces, pictures, actions, gestures and signs, but ill-suited for verbal learning. This is not to deny that beyond early childhood, many of us prefer to learn visually from books. Research studies, however, indicate that verbal material, whether spoken or written, is filtered through our auditory and articulatory coding system.

Characteristics and Limitations
of a Guided Interactional Approach

In this chapter we have attempted to describe our approach to language development for the hearing-impaired child. We have drawn from the accumulated knowledge of past centuries, both consciously and unconsciously, and make no claim to the method's uniqueness or universal applicability. Certainly, in the absence of the various prerequisite conditions laid forth in the first chapter, fluent spoken language is an unrealistic goal for profoundly hearing-impaired children. Even under good conditions, certain children may fail to learn spoken language. However, if ongoing assessment is the rule, such children will be identified readily and alternative programs arranged.

The basic principles are:

1. The social interaction between parent and child is the basis for the development of vocal communication followed by verbal communication.

2. The normal developmental stages of child language acquisition should be followed as closely as possible.

3. Parent-infant communication must be guided and monitored in such a way as to permit optimal reception of speech (via audition, vision, and touch).

4. The child's auditory-vocal and later his auditory-verbal skills must be guided and monitored.

5. The form and content of the language used by the parent must be monitored and guided so that it is tailored to the child's psychological needs and his linguistic level.

Possible reasons for limited progress in the development of spoken language include damage to the child's central nervous system or, specifically, to the language area of the brain. More often, the cause is to be found elsewhere: perhaps an unremarked progressive hearing impairment, unsuitable or malfunctioning hearing aids, inadequate use of residual hearing, failure to develop motor speech skills through babble, poor parental cooperation or failure to understand the program goals, faulty environmental conditions, or an inadequately trained teacher.

The following are approximate guidelines relating to progress.

1. Progress in listening and vocalizing (as per A. H. Ling's *Schedules of Development*, 1977) should be evidenced within the first three months. If absent, comprehensive assessment procedures should be undertaken.

2. Alertness to sound and the production of syllabic babble should appear within 6 months. Auditory and/or visual attention to speech should be achieved.

3. The beginnings of language comprehension and the use of

word approximations should be noted somewhere between 6 and 12 months after training has begun.

4. Two-word combinations should occur after about 2 years of training.

5. Sentences with a subject and predicate should be used no later than 3 years from the beginning of training.

When progress is slower than normal, or if there is little noticeable progress after 12 months of training, the following procedures are recommended:

1. Comprehensive re-evaluation in all areas of development by a team of specialists.

2. Thorough check of hearing aids and their suitability.

3. Assessment of parent-child as well as child-parent communication.

4. Frank discussion with the parents of the findings of the assessment team.

5. Revision of the program in consultation with the parents, with special attention to ensure that the prerequisite conditions for the learning of spoken language are met. Possibilities include compensating for deterioration of hearing (visual or tactile cues may be introduced or new hearing aids obtained), provision of increased individual attention from a highly skilled teacher/clinician (two or three times weekly, rather than once), and/or psychological counseling for the parents.

6. Reassessment and revision of goals within three months of the new program.

If progress continues to be slow, and the child is at least 3 years old, daily attendance (half-days for 3- and 4-year-olds) at a child-centered program is probably appropriate (see Chapter 13). Parent guidance should be maintained on a once-weekly basis. Teacher/clinicians will have to work hard to ensure that the hearing-impaired child can experience ample one-to-one interaction in which language can best be learned, and that he has lots of contact with normal-hearing and talking peers. The danger of a segregated setting is that the child will be exposed to poor speech and language models from his peers and that nonverbal child-to-child communication will predominate.

As long as spoken language is the primary goal, introduction of the written form should be delayed until the child is producing sentences with a subject and predicate, and has reached a mental age of 5 or 6 years. For children who can produce two- or three-word phrases but who cannot formulate simple sentences by age 6 or 7 years, a carefully structured program, such as that utilized by McGrath, Nicholls, and Truscott (1977) is recommended. This is an area in which considerable research is required.

If very little or no progress in spoken language development can be measured, and the various prerequisite conditions have been met, the child should be transferred to a program emphasizing sign language. A period of 18–24 months of training under a highly skilled teacher/clinician should be more than adequate to indicate whether or not a hearing-impaired child has the potential to develop spoken language. For a multi-handicapped child, a slower rate of progress would be expected, but if no progress has been made in the acquisition of spoken language after 18–24 months, an alternative communication system is urgently needed.

Initial emphasis on whatever the child's auditory capacity will have the advantage of orienting him to acoustic cues which will facilitate behaviors crucial for the acquisition of spoken language: attending when spoken to, extending his vocal repertoire, attaching meaning to intonation and phonetic patterns, and using first, vocal and, later, verbal communication.

Precise knowledge of the structure of spoken language is crucial if the hearing-impaired child is to progress academically. Verbal reasoning depends on knowing the finer points of the language. It is, therefore, our view that every effort should be made to ensure that all hearing-impaired children are at least given the chance to learn spoken language first, and with that as a basis, reading and writing.

ANNOTATED BIBLIOGRAPHY

Blackwell, P., Engen, E., Fischgrund, J. E., and Zarcadoolas, C. *Sentences and Other Systems: A Language and Learning Curriculum for Hearing-Impaired Children.* Washington, D.C.: The A. G. Bell Association for the Deaf, 1978.
This new text, based on the Rhode Island School for the Deaf Curriculum Guide, describes an approach to language development which emphasizes initial focus on five basic sentence patterns. Language development and curriculum outlines for preschool through high school are presented, with the written form being introduced as early as age 3. The reader will find an excellent review of the normal processes of cognitive and linguistic development in the early chapters.

Crystal, D., Fletcher, P., and Garman, M. *The Grammatical Analysis of Language Disability: A Procedure for Assessment and Remediation.* London, England: Arnold, 1976.
The language assessment procedure described in this book consists of the analysis of a half-hour sample of spoken language which can be utilized with children or adults. A profile chart showing developmental stages is provided, and two case studies are presented to illustrate assessment and remedial procedures. The focus is on syntax: A knowledge of psycholinguistics is essential.

Dale, D. M. C. *Language Development in Deaf and Partially Hearing Children.* Springfield, Ill.: Charles C Thomas, 1974.
Dale reviews methods of language teaching utilized by teachers of the hearing-impaired in special schools, classes, and units in regular schools. He stresses the importance of individual teaching. A large part of the book is devoted to the presentation of language topics for children aged 3 to 17 years. Of interest to students, teacher/clinicians, and parents.

Ewing, A. W. G., and Ewing, E. C. *Teaching Deaf Children To Talk.* Manchester, England: University Press, 1964 (formerly available from the Volta Bureau).
This is one of many books written by the Ewings, who have contributed greatly to the education of hearing-impaired children. They advocate a developmental approach to language development for hearing-impaired infants and young children through parent guidance. For older children, they recommend an approach which combines listening, reading, and speaking.

Fitzgerald, E.   *Straight Language for the Deaf.* Washington, D.C.: The Volta Bureau, 1949; 18th printing, 1976.

This book describes a system of language instruction involving keywords and symbols. It is popularly known as the Fitzgerald Key because the question headings, *who, what, where, when, how, why,* were considered to be the key by which deaf children could be taught to formulate correct English sentences and to think verbally. Direct teaching by a grammatical approach, with the written form as the medium of instruction, was seen to be essential because of the absence of audition and the limitations of the speechread pattern. It appeared as early as 1929 at a time when little use could be made of residual hearing, and when preschool training was rare. The method still has its adherents, few of whom apply it with the flexibility intended by the author.

Groht, M. A.   *Natural Language for Deaf Children.* Washington, D.C.: The A. G. Bell Association for the Deaf, 1958; 8th printing, 1977.

Although Mildred Groht and Edith Fitzgerald were both master teachers and had essentially the same goals for deaf children, their methods were quite different. Groht considered that language could and should be learned through oral communication. The teacher was expected to use whatever language was natural and appropriate to the situation, following no set order in introducing verb tenses or sentence patterns. Language was developed through speechreading in the preschool, with the written form as a supplement by age 5. This approach depends on the teacher's knowledge of normal child language and skill in stimulating oral communication.

Harris, G. M.   *Language for the Preschool Deaf Child.* New York: Grune and Stratton, third edition, 1971.

Teachers and parents of preschool hearing-impaired children will enjoy learning from the author's many years of experience. The text reflects a strong orientation to the use of vision as well as hearing. Children receive an early exposure to the printed form. Over 100 lessons are provided, each containing suggestions for sense training, lipreading, speech and auditory training.

Jacobovits, L. A., and Gordon, B.   *The Context of Foreign Language Teaching.* Rowley, Mass.: Newbury House Publishers Inc., 1974.

Teachers of hearing-impaired children of elementary and high-school age will find a fascinating and helpful discussion of the problems of language teaching. The authors stress that communicative skills are best developed when the learner participates regularly in social situations where person-to-person interaction is compelling. The transactional aspects of conversations are analyzed to demonstrate how fluency in a language involves much more than the ability to produce grammatically correct sentences.

Lee, L. L. *Developmental Sentence Analysis.* Evanston, Ill.: Northwestern University Press, 1974.

The author presents a grammatical assessment procedure, based on the analysis of a language sample. The text is intended for speech and language clinicians working with language-delayed children and provides guidelines for devising suitable training programs. Readers are provided with background information on psycholinguistics. Further details are included in the chapter preceding this bibliography.

Lee, L. L., Koenigsknecht, R. A., and Mulhern, S. *Interactive Language Development Teaching.* Evanston, Ill.: Northwestern University Press, 1975.

The authors describe a clinical technique for assisting children to improve the grammatical structure of their spoken language. The intent is to simulate the verbal interchange between parent and child through the use of brief stories written in the form of conversations. The language of the stories follows the graded developmental progression described in Lee's Developmental Sentence Analysis. Student teacher/clinicians will find this book helpful.

Ling, D., and Ling, A. H. *Basic Vocabulary and Language Thesaurus for Hearing-Impaired Children.* Washington, D.C.: The A. G. Bell Association for the Deaf, 1977.

More than 2,000 words are listed by topic, according to their frequency of usage by young normal-hearing children. Common phrases and expressions are also provided. Included are sections on question forms with typical answers and verbs—strong, weak, and auxiliary. Written for parents and teacher/clinicians working with young children.

Lloyd, L. L. (Ed.) *Communication Assessment and Intervention Strategies.* Baltimore, Md.: University Park Press, 1976.

A comprehensive text aimed at professionals working with a variety of communication disorders. Teacher/clinicians will find a useful discussion of Language Assessment by G. M. Siegel and P. A. Broen. There are several appendices including Rules of Talking, one which provides details on various Language Assessment Procedures, and one on Language Intervention Systems available in kit form.

McGrath, G., Nicholls, G., and Truscott, I.   Teaching language to hearing-impaired children of school age. *Australian Teacher of the Deaf*, 18, 14–21, 1977.

These authors present a rationale and brief outline of a language program designed to teach the structures of English through a controlled interchange between teacher and pupils. It is based on the Tate Oral English Course (see Tate) developed for Pacific Islands children. The aim is to develop precise verbal thinking through the accurate use of English. This approach would appear to have something to offer to teachers working with hearing-impaired children who have reached age 7 without mastering the essentials of spoken English. However, a comprehensive account of the authors' adaptation of the Tate program would be required.

Merson, R. M., Fishman, B. V., and Fowler, S. A. (Eds.)   *Central Institute Test Evaluation Booklet*. Cedar Falls, Iowa: Go-Mo Industries, Inc., 1976.

Teacher/clinicians will find this booklet helpful in informing them about a variety of speech and language tests. Comments are provided under Purpose, Description, Materials, Age Range, Administration and Scoring, Norms, Reliability, Clinical Assets, Clinical Liabilities, Address for Ordering, Cost, and Relevant References.

Russell, W. K., Quigley, S. P., and Power, D. J.   *Linguistics and Deaf Children*. Washington, D.C.: The A. G. Bell Association for the Deaf, 1976.

A technical book for those with some knowledge of psycholinguistics. Of particular interest to classroom teachers of hearing-impaired children are the sections toward the end of each chapter. Here one finds details of the structures which create most difficulty for hearing-impaired children, together with notes on normal acquisition. Analysis of a popular series of readers reveals their unsuitability for children with impoverished language.

Tate, G. M.   *Oral English.* Wellington, N.Z.: A. H. and A. W. Reed, 182 Wakefield St., 1971.

This handbook provides an overview of the Tate Oral English Course utilized by McGrath et al (see bibliography). The course consists of 15 books which cover the teaching of the many structured elements of English in a systematic way. These are the very elements which create confusion for so many hearing-impaired children. The oral course is backed up by controlled readers designed for children growing up in the Pacific Islands.

Tyack, D., and Gottsleben, R.   *Language Sampling, Analysis and Training.* Palo Alto, Calif.: Consulting Psychologists Press, 1974.

This is a handbook for teacher/clinicians which describes procedures for sampling and analyzing language, for writing behavioral training programs, and for recording and reporting information. The analysis and training focus on syntax acquisition for children with mean sentence lengths between two and six words. Although the techniques are very clearly described, a basic knowledge of psycholinguistics is required.

van Uden, A.   *A World of Language for Deaf Children.* Amsterdam and Lisse: Swets and Zeitlinger, 3rd edition, 1977.

The author favors a conversational as opposed to a formal, grammatical approach to language development. The teacher is expected to take the role of the mother and attempt to express what the child wishes to say, providing him with both question and answer if necessary. The author believes that access to the written form of such conversations will assist the hearing-impaired child to deduce the rules of language.

12.   Language and Reading

*T*here is complete agreement among professionals that ability to read and write English is of the greatest importance to hearing-impaired children. There is considerable disagreement, however, on how to achieve literacy. Traditional techniques have not succeeded with a large proportion of children.

Although it is recognized that the normal-hearing child is a fluent speaker of his native tongue before he is ever taught to read, many teachers consider that the hearing-impaired child will benefit from early exposure to the written form. The reason given is that only imperfect patterns are available through speechreading and residual hearing and therefore the written form should be presented in order to provide the child with the "complete" pattern, which in turn will enable him to understand sentence structures. Such reasoning is equivalent to saying that by providing native English speakers with the written form of Arabic, we could readily master its syntax. There is nothing magical about the written form. The underlying meaning is not self-evident. It has to be learned.

It is tempting for teachers of hearing-impaired children to introduce the written form to children as young as 3 or 4 years, since many of them are quite capable of learning to associate a printed label with a given object. A vocabulary of 50 to 100 nouns and 10 to 15 verbs may be taught quite quickly in this manner. It provides evidence that the teacher is able to teach and the child is able to learn. Such results may be impressive in the short term, but they tend to provide a false sense of confidence in the child's mastery of language. The 5-year-old hearing-impaired child may even appear to be more advanced in this respect than his normal-hearing counterpart who has not yet had any instruction in reading. For the hearing-impaired child, the hundred or so words that he can recognize in their printed form may constitute his total (written and spoken) vocabulary, whereas by age 5 the normal-hearing child is likely to have a spoken vocabulary of somewhere between 3,000 and 5,000 words. In addition, he has control over the basic sentence structures of spoken English. His comprehension and use of his native language permit him to make deductions and inferences about the meaning of written language.

The normal-hearing child takes a year or two to master the mechanical aspects of reading, that is, the discovery of the relationships between the spoken and written forms of his language. As soon as these relationships are known, his education can progress in leaps and bounds, since he is in a position to gain information from books. The typical reading primers contain no information whatsoever. They merely provide the child with practice in converting print to sound and sound to meaning. Following sufficient practice the child becomes able to perceive the meaning directly from the printed form.

Preparation for Reading

Before Reading

Although we deplore the early teaching of reading to hearing-impaired children or, for that matter, to their normal-hearing peers, we are convinced of the value as well as the pleasure to be obtained from introducing children to the world of books as early as 9 or 10 months of age. The normal-hearing baby enjoys the colors and textures of books made of cloth or very hard board and the experience of being held on someone's lap while he listens to what is said about the pictures. If the book contains nursery rhymes, he enjoys hearing them sung. When he is by himself, he will babble and sing to himself, turning the pages and patting the pictures. From about 12 to 15 months he will begin to recognize pictures of familiar objects or people and will gleefully point to them when asked. At first he will want to turn the pages quickly, looking only briefly at each picture. Gradually, he will look more attentively at the pictures and will begin noticing details, recognizing one object after another and appreciating the actions which are depicted.

The hearing-impaired baby also benefits greatly from such early experiences with books. There is no need to have him face the speaker or for him to be trained to look back and forth between the picture book and the speaker's face. Rather, he should sit on his mother's (or someone else's) lap, snuggled closely against the reader's body. He is thus positioned optimally for auditory reception, since the speaker's mouth will be only a few inches from the microphone of his hearing aids. Thus, from early childhood, the hearing-impaired youngster can learn to gain pleasure from books—to interpret pictures; to understand that spoken words can be related to what he sees in pictures; to use words and phrases to describe what he sees in books; to ask questions about what he sees; and to think about related ideas which are not illustrated. "Read book" will become a favorite cry. In imitation of his parents and older siblings, he too will sit down with a book and "read."

Before Writing

Scribbling permits the child to develop visual-motor control, to attend to the variety of shapes and lines that can be created and at the same time amuse himself. One-year-old babies make marks on paper, if given a thick crayon, and by 20 months they scribble vigorously. Shortly after their second birthday they can draw horizontal and vertical strokes, at first by imitation and then by copying. By age 3, they can make primitive drawings of a circle and a cross. Ability not only to recognize but also to produce such differences prepares the child for distinguishing visual aspects of printed words, which will, in turn, lead him to identify words and letters. Between the ages of 3 and 5 years, and without tuition, the child's scribbling becomes more deliberate. One can distinguish his pictures from his "writing." The writing varies in height, and spaces appear as they do between words—resembling whatever models are available to the child. Actual letters begin to be formed. Scribbling and babbling permit an apprenticeship period in which the visual-motor or auditory-speech-motor skills can be developed before the child has the capacity for symbolic activity.

Parents of a hearing-impaired child should ensure that he has lots of opportunity to scribble and to draw. Some parents are reluctant to permit such activity in case their child should draw on walls or tabletops. From the beginning, children should be supervised when scribbling or chalking. The child should be shown where and how such activities may take place. He should never be allowed to scribble on story books or to tear or spoil books of any sort. A hearing-impaired child can easily be brought to understand the rules, and pencils and books should be removed immediately if he attempts to misuse them. If he is clearly shown how to use and enjoy them, there should not be any problem.

Personal Factors Related to Reading

Persistence in figuring out how to do things is an important prerequisite skill for the beginning reader. The making of jigsaw puzzles is an activity through which the child can develop confidence in working at a project, first by trial and error, and later by some sort of strategy. Instead of selecting the appropriate piece for the child, his mother can provide verbal cues, such as "Turn it around," "Look for the boy's head," or "Find a green piece." She can also praise him for trying and help him finish the puzzle, if necessary. In learning to read, the child must have confidence in himself and in his ability to do things or to ask for information or help on occasion. He should not be afraid of making errors, and should be made aware that most people, including his parents, are prone to error from time to time.

To be successful, a beginning reader should have a mental age of about 5 years, in addition to abundant language and pre-reading experience. It is better to delay reading instruction than to introduce it too early in order to avoid frustration of both teacher and child.

Beginning Reading

The child who is able to talk and who begins to produce recognizable letters, will spontaneously ask, usually about age 5, what letters are called and what words say. He has become aware that print conveys meaning, since adults and older children can tell stories based on the written form. The normal-hearing child whose parents have read to him, told him stories, and sung him songs will almost certainly, by age 5, have a repertoire of stories and songs that he can recall from memory. Earlier, he would probably have been prompted to recite parts of a rhyme or story and would have been reinforced for his attempts.

Without guidance, the parents of a hearing-impaired child are likely to provide him with relatively little in the way of storytelling or singing simply because of their awareness that he cannot hear.

Part of the problem, of course, could be that without amplification and unable to understand what is said, the hearing-impaired child finds little of interest in the storytelling situation. He probably prefers to look at picture books by himself. Parents of a hearing-impaired child should be shown how they can exploit time spent with books as an avenue first, to spoken, and later, to written language. Time should be set aside each day—perhaps after a midmorning snack, and again before bedtime—for Mom or Dad to "read" a story.

Dramatic interpretations of stories will be much appreciated. To provide necessary contrast the reader can produce a gruff voice for Father Bear, a melodious voice for Mother Bear, and a squeaky voice for Baby Bear. Somewhat exaggerated intonation patterns can be used to advantage in such questions as "Who's been sitting on my chair?" By such action, parents can help extend the range of the child's auditory linguistic experience and help develop auditory memory by lending more salience and excitement to the process of linking the written and spoken forms.

The hearing-impaired child should be encouraged to tell his version of the story. Exact repetition is not especially desirable, for the child's command of spoken language will be enhanced by his being able to describe the actions freely in his own words. He should be given the opportunity to discover that there are many acceptable ways of expressing a particular idea. The ability to paraphrase—an essential part of verbal learning—can thus be developed through spoken language. Paraphrasing of written language should not then create the headaches it does for the hearing-impaired child who learns language principally through its written form.

Flexibility is hindered when language is presented and developed from the written form as early as the nursery school years, for the child learns stereotyped forms. When an activity is described on an experience chart simple sentence by simple sentence and is rehearsed from the same written form day after day, the hearing-impaired child is likely to deduce that only these words or sentence patterns are appropriate. If he deviates from them, perhaps by omitting or mispronouncing a word, he often is told he is wrong and his attention is drawn to the chart.

If the purpose of the experience chart is to present complete models of English sentences and provide practice in their use, why not repeat the activity itself, or conduct another activity which will draw upon the same vocabulary and sentence patterns? If the written form is used, it should be provided anew on each occasion. A better alternative is to ask the children to reconstruct, orally, the events which took place. The child can be prompted from a series of drawings made either by the teacher, the parent, or the child himself immediately following the experience. In this way, there can be discussion not only of the events as they happened, but of other related ideas which he should be encouraged to express.

Methods of Beginning Reading Instruction

It is quite a common practice to teach normal-hearing preschool children the names of the letters of the alphabet and their sequence. If is often assumed that knowledge of the letter names is essential to beginning reading, but this is not so. Letter names are required for oral spelling and are helpful for story-writing, but they should be learned gradually and incidentally as the children become interested. The letters occurring in their names should be learned first.

For hearing-impaired children at the preschool level, deliberate teaching of the letter names as a first step in reading is harmful. The child is likely to be confused because the names of the letters do not correspond with their sounds. It is a formidable task for the young hearing-impaired child to identify and recall the names of 26 unrelated items. The alphabet song is not likely to assist him greatly because of the difficulty of articulating the letter names. Time spent in such an activity would be much better used in developing the child's linguistic skills.

There are two major approaches to the teaching of reading, the phonic method and the whole-word or look-and-say method.

The Phonic Method

In the phonic method, the child learns the sounds made by the letters, and the hope is that this process will help him identify the spoken equivalents of words. Preparation for this task includes practice in listening for particular sounds in words. For example, the child is asked to find a word beginning with the sound [s], or to pick out the word that does not begin with [s] from a set of several that do. Current research indicates that it is not until age 6 or 7 that the majority of normal-hearing children are able to segment words into their phonetic components, an analytic task which requires high-level cognitive abilities. This approach is much less suitable for English than for a language like Spanish, which has fairly regular letter-to-sound correspondances.

For the hearing-impaired child, especially if he does not have perfect speech, the phonic method is particularly unsuitable in the early stages. He is taught that the letter "b" says [bə], "a" says [æ] and "t" says [tə]. Blending such sounds together produces [bəætə], rather than /bæt/. Such an approach is detrimental to speech production (see Chapter 10) as well as to reading. Regular teachers who have hearing-impaired children in their classes would be well-advised to begin with a whole-word approach (see below), delaying the teaching of phonic skills until the child has acquired a good sight vocabulary and can produce most speech sounds clearly.

"Sounding out" a word is supposed to help the child use the auditory pattern as a way of referring to his long-term memory store of words. This strategy is only likely to help the hearing-impaired child who has good residual audition and clear speech and who, therefore, like his normal-hearing peers, uses auditory and articulatory coding in short-term memory. He should then be able to retrieve matching words and their meanings from his long-term memory store. Sounding out a word is only of help if that word is already part of the child's spoken vocabulary. It is of no help with new words unless they are related to known words such as "farm" and "farmer."

Another problem of the phonic approach is that by focusing the child's attention first upon the surface character of the word, one directs him to a letter-by-letter strategy and distracts him from the real purpose of reading, which is to extract meaning from print. Such a tactic discourages the child from utilizing the linguistic context to assist him in decoding an unfamiliar written form.

The Whole Word Method

The whole word, or look-and-say, method is probably the most suitable for beginning reading whether the child is normal-hearing or hearing-impaired. It involves a direct association between the written and spoken word and between the written word and its referent. This approach can be combined with another method, which involves the identification of whole sentences.

Individual words from the child's spoken vocabulary can be printed on flash cards, and the child can learn to respond quickly and automatically with the spoken equivalent. He should also learn to write words and letters, and to match them or indicate which one of a set is different. He will thus become increasingly attentive to the appearance of individual letters.

The hearing-impaired child should have a concurrent speech development program through which he will become able to produce syllables such as "bee" (B), "see" (C), "kay" (K), and "eff" (F), or "at," "cat," "sat," and "fat." He will then have little difficulty in learning the names and sounds of the letters of the alphabet or in following a program in phonics somewhat later.

The first words to be learned should be those of special interest to the particular child, e.g., his name, "Mommy," "Daddy," and the names of his friends. Other words should look and sound very different—"airplane," "car," and "truck," for example. The 5-year-old child finds it relatively easy to recognize words from their overall pattern and he takes note of their initial and final letters. The ability to recognize words gives him immediate satisfaction, and he develops confidence that he is able to learn to read.

Given the complicated nature of English spellings and the large number of very common words which are not pronounced according to simple rules, it makes sense to develop a sizeable word recognition vocabulary before introducing phonics. Many of the common words which are exceptions to the phonic rules should be taught by sight. Examples of such words are "is," "was," "have," and "come." Of course, if the child is to have some means of discovering how to read new words from their written form at a later stage, he should be helped to develop word attack skills through phonics.

The key to progress beyond the word identification stage of reading is familiarity with the vocabulary and syntactic structures of English. A brief glance at early readers will reveal that even if the hearing-impaired child is able to recognize the words, there is no guarantee that he will comprehend the sentences in which they occur.

If the hearing-impaired child is to be sufficiently motivated to learn to read, he must experience success in comprehending the material in his early readers. In the beginning, every word and sentence should be understood in its spoken form before it is presented in writing. The hearing-impaired child will then experience the thrill of discovering that he too can read, *read* in the real sense of understanding. Teachers and parents may therefore find it necessary to make the child's first reading books.

These home-made books can be prepared with the child's current interests in mind. He might enjoy providing some of the illustrations himself and even, with help, supply the wording of the text. The parent or teacher can do the actual printing. Books which the child has helped to prepare will become cherished possessions and will be read over and over again. Sometimes he will read them for his own pleasure. At other times he will proudly display his newly acquired skills to any willing listener.

Suitability of Available Readers

One of the major benefits of following a basal reading series is that the vocabulary is carefully controlled, ensuring that new words are repeated several times throughout the book and are included for review later in the series. Unfortunately, most current basal readers were prepared by persons unaware of recent psycholinguistic developments. The result is the inclusion of syntactic structures which are beyond the comprehension of the normal-hearing beginning reader, and consequently far beyond that of the hearing-impaired child.

For maximum impact, the learner should be able to read each of his early books in one sitting. The sense of satisfaction in reading an *entire* book is enormous. It is unreasonable to expect a child to maintain interest in a story when he reads it a little at a time over a period of days, or weeks. The child should read a different little book each day. One way to provide this experience is to cut up existing readers which contain a series of short stories. An attractive cover can be made for each booklet. The child will be delighted to take such booklets home to read to various members of his family. He may also enjoy keeping a record of the number of books he can read.

Teachers and parents may encounter difficulty in locating suitable texts for older hearing-impaired children who have limited spoken language and reading skills. It is crucial that the interest level is appropriate for the particular child; otherwise he will make little attempt to learn to read. Once again, home-made books related to hobbies and sports may be part of the answer. Information about specially written texts for older slow readers can be obtained from various publishers, including the A. G. Bell

Association for the Deaf. Details are also available in the texts by Hart and by Schonell and Goodacre (see bibliography).

Oral Reading

With young normal-hearing children, oral reading is the predominant means of early instruction, and children take turns at reading aloud. This procedure helps the teacher to discover which children are able to retrieve the spoken from the written form. If a child is able to read a passage orally, the teacher will tend to assume that he is able to understand what he has read. Class lessons of oral reading are painful for both good and poor readers.

Group oral reading lessons are quite unsuitable for hearing-impaired children because of wide individual differences in hearing levels, speech, language, and reading. The reading skills of a hearing-impaired child are unlikely to be developed while he sits and attempts to follow a classmate's poorly articulated rendition of the printed material. Although the small size of special classes permits individual teaching, even then a reading lesson should not become the vehicle for speech and language teaching. When the hearing-impaired child has to read aloud he has to undertake several processes simultaneously, none of which he has developed to an automatic level. He has to comprehend the syntactic and semantic aspects, and then think about how to pronounce the words. When the fluent reader reads aloud, his eye travels ahead of his voice. If it is a single sentence, he takes in the meaning before he begins to articulate the words. He is then able to read aloud with expression. Someone who is unfamiliar with the language will tend to process each word separately, stumbling over the pronunciation and making it difficult for listeners to grasp the meaning. If he is asked to read a paragraph, rather than a sentence, he will probably have difficulty in remembering what it contained. His attention has had to be focused on articulation.

Research indicates that, in the case of hearing-impaired children with poor speech, their comprehension of material is hindered by oral reading. Parents and teachers of hearing-impaired children should therefore be sparing in their use of oral reading except where a child speaks fluently and automatically.

Reading and Listening

Children with moderate spoken language skills can be aided by listening to a good reader. The material can be tape-recorded and presented through headphones, the written form being available for the child to follow visually, while he listens. In the early stages, the content should be thoroughly familiar to the child, and the words should be in his reading vocabulary. The recording may be the recounting of an experience in which the child has taken part; it may be based on familiar routines; it could be a traditional story; or, with older children, a part of a geography or history unit. The young child enjoys the inclusion of sound effects, and the use of different voices for the narrator and the various characters.

Listening and reading is one way of making reading a pleasurable experience. Material can be prepared to suit individual children. If the story is tape-recorded, one child may listen while the teacher works with another. At any time, the teacher can stop the tape recorder and ask the child to indicate on the book or typescript which sentence has just been read. The child can also be asked to tell the story to classmates or to a member of his family.

Parents can read aloud to their children from books in which the material is slightly more advanced than those which the child can read unaided. The child can follow the print and enjoy the story and learn a small number of new words and phrases through the context of the story. The child can enjoy longer stories, can be stimulated by thought-provoking ideas, and can acquire factual information when he is not under pressure to read such material aloud or on his own.

Language Enrichment To Facilitate Reading

Even after the hearing-impaired child has mastered the early stages of reading, he will continue to benefit from a program which emphasizes language enrichment, rather than reading instruction. Research has indicated that hearing-impaired children in special schools have language deficiencies which prevent them from understanding even the early readers. Restricted vocabularies are common even among children with mild to moderate hearing impairment. The major deficiency is in relation to the comprehension of syntactic structures. Among hearing-impaired children, the verbs "is" and "has" are commonly used interchangeably; the reference of pronouns is poorly understood; question forms, particularly those introduced by auxiliary verbs such as "can," "is," and "does" cause problems, as does the use of the passive voice. A sentence such as "The boy was hit by the girl" is often mistakenly processed as "The boy hit the girl." The sentence "He went to school after he had lunch" may be understood as being equivalent to "He went to school and had lunch afterwards."

Teachers and parents should consider it a wise investment of time to ensure that their children are familiar with the sentence structures which will occur in future reading books. Good spoken language can be developed by following a guided interactional program such as that described in the previous chapter.

The hearing-impaired child has difficulties which are similar to those of a person attempting to read a foreign language. The regular classroom teacher and certainly the parent should reflect from his own experience. Word knowledge does not guarantee sentence comprehension. The overall meaning of a paragraph may be unclear when one has had to work out the meaning of each sentence, little by little, for one's memory becomes overburdened. This is also true for the hearing-impaired child. The fluent reader can skim through a book or article written in his native language. The person with less than native skill is obliged to read every word in order to extract the meaning, and even then he may make grave errors. An adult is unlikely to read a foreign-language book for pleasure, unless it is effortless. If he has to use a dictionary frequently, reading becomes labored and comprehension is reduced. Vocabulary and syntax have to be 99 percent familiar for reading to be enjoyable.

Spoken language can be greatly enriched through games, for language learned in "fun" situations is retained without difficulty. The child is barely aware that his parents and teachers are intent on language development when his attention is absorbed in a game. Bright 2-year-olds and average 3-year-olds will enjoy picture dominoes, and 4- and 5-year-olds will have fun playing all kinds of dice games which will simultaneously develop number concepts and social behavior. The older the child, of course, the more complicated can be the game. Card games provide lots of variety. Most children enjoy card tricks and magic and should be encouraged to perform their skills. Checkers leads on to chess. The child can learn all the phrases appropriate to each game and also learn to think and plan. Games involving language skill and general knowledge appeal to the older child. Teachers might even think of suggesting games rather than the more usual homework assignments.

Reading, Writing, and Spelling

Earlier in this chapter we described how looking at books, on the one hand, and scribbling, on the other, can help to prepare the child for reading and writing. Reading and writing are indeed complementary skills. Word recognition is facilitated by the child's being able to produce the word in its written form. The hearing-impaired child should be encouraged, but not forced, to copy words and sentences which he can understand and read.

In imitation of his teacher, the young child will want to label his drawings or write about an experience. As soon as the child shows a spontaneous desire to write about his own interests, he should be helped to do so. If he wants to send a letter to Grandma, his mother should first write to his dictation, keeping as close as possible to the spoken forms he uses. Before long, he will want to write "all by himself" but will require assistance with spelling. By this time, he can be taught the names of any letters he has not yet learned.

We have found it advantageous to teach spelling in a systematic way once the child has reached about a grade 2 reading level, and while he is learning phonics. For children with good articulation, learning to spell provides practice in listening and speaking, as well as in writing the words. This procedure also encourages auditory and articulatory coding as part of the memory process. For children with poor articulation, spelling should be taught through vision. Parents should ensure that the meanings of the words have been taught well ahead of time. Parents can provide the child with sentences in which the words to be learned are used.

In our experience, Schonell's *Essentials of Teaching and Testing Spelling* (see bibliography) cannot be bettered. It includes 3,200 words to be learned over a five-year period. The words are presented in families so that children are helped to derive the rules of English spelling. For 7-year-olds, the weekly assignment is 12 words. Three words are to be learned each night, Monday through Thursday, and the entire set is reviewed for Friday's test. Here is an example:

date	be	fine	mate
hate	free	pine	case
plate	queen	shine	chase

This approach has an excellent rationale, in contrast to the common practice of selecting unrelated words from the child's reading books. Words which are easy to read are not necessarily those which are easy to spell, and some words which are easy to spell ("was" and "saw," "no" and "on") may be confused by inexperienced readers.

Language and Education

Parents or regular classroom teachers may be surprised to discover that hearing-impaired children have difficulty in subjects other than reading or English. However, even very early math concepts depend on the child's understanding of the language used. For example, "John has 4 apples and Bill gave him 2 more." does not mean the same as "John has 4 apples and Bill has 2 more."

Parents can do a great deal to prepare their hearing-impaired child to understand the spoken and written language of numbers and math. Experiences with sand and water can be used to develop notions of "full" and "empty," "half-full," "too much," and "more." For further suggestions see *Basic Vocabulary and Language Thesaurus for Hearing-Impaired Children* (Ling & Ling, 1977).

At more advanced levels, the child needs language for reasoning, "If . . . , then . . . ," "What will happen if . . . ". The learning of science, geography, history, and social studies—in fact, any form of verbal learning—depends on the child being able to understand his textbooks. Textbooks are difficult even for normal-hearing students when the subject is new, and there is a great deal of special terminology introduced with minimal explanation. Markedly greater problems are experienced by hearing-impaired students because of the increasingly complex sentence structures used. Parents and teachers should plan well ahead so that the hearing-impaired child is familiar with the vocabulary and sentence structures when he comes to read them.

Reading as a Means To Facilitate Language Growth

It is only after the hearing-impaired child has a good grasp of spoken language and has mastered the mechanics of reading that he will be in a position to develop his language through reading. Furthermore, he is only likely to attempt to learn through reading if it is not a frustrating experience. The material should be at least 95 percent familiar to him. The child who comprehends a wide range of syntactic structures will be able to guess the meaning of new words and even idiomatic expressions from the wider context of the sentence or paragraph. Parents and teachers should therefore be prepared to expend considerable effort in locating or creating books and materials which their children can read and enjoy on their own.

The hearing-impaired child should be exposed to books on all sorts of topics, since books can open up new worlds of interest for the child from the earliest stages. Children enjoy real life stories, fairy tales, poetry, wildlife, sports, and hobbies. As the child's reading skills develop, the more he can gain from books. Self-motivated reading can often be promoted through comics because so much of the story is carried by illustrations. Although illustrated books are always a delight, fewer and fewer illustrations are essential to comprehension as the child's language and reading skills increase.

Basic Guidelines for Parents

The following points summarize the main ideas expressed in this chapter as they concern parents.

1. You should not attempt to teach reading to hearing-impaired children before they are speaking spontaneously in simple phrases. The words used in the first readers should be a part of their spoken vocabulary. In later stages, children will be able to learn new vocabulary and language through reading, but not initially. In initial reading, the child should be allowed to concentrate his attention on the learning of one thing—not a new word, but how to recognize the written form of a word he already uses in its spoken form.

2. Low standards of reading among hearing-impaired children are partly caused by a too-early start on reading. The task is

much too difficult for 3- or 4-year-old children—particularly for those with limited speech and language.

3. The child's speech should be clear enough to allow him to say intelligibly all the words that appear in his first reading books.

4. If hearing is present, auditory discrimination should be well enough developed to permit the child to hear the reading vocabulary and to discriminate between the words used.

5. Before reading is begun, visual discrimination should be developed to the point which allows the child to match (a) picture to picture, (b) word to word and picture, (c) sentence to sentence and picture, and (d) letter to letter.

6. Innate ability and past experience of the child largely determine whether a child is ready for reading. Some children have specific disabilities which hold back their reading progress. While, in general, only the teacher should teach the child to read, parents can do much to encourage the acquisition of reading skills and to promote an interest in reading.

7. Before early reading books can be successfully used, the child should be able to interpret pictures they contain. He should be able to see what they are about and to express this in phrases, spontaneously or with the help of leading questions. The main point of the picture should be elicited first by questions such as "Tell me about the picture," "What is the boy doing?", "What happened to the dog?", and "What do you think the boy said?". Questions that can be answered with "yes" or "no" are of limited value in developing language.

At the early reading stage the child is already able to answer "What's that?" and other simple questions. There is no need to discuss "How many?" or "What color?" unless these relate to the central idea of the picture. Too often these questions are used to the exclusion of other, more important, ones. This practice can lead to the child missing the main theme and being at a disadvantage when it comes to dealing with questions which are not answered directly in the text. This can be a major problem with older children who have not been encouraged to think about what they are reading.

8. A child is really ready to read when he begins to ask, "What does that word say?", "Tell me what it says under the picture," "Read the words," etc. He really looks at the print and wants to follow word for word as you read. You should never read one

word at a time. This destroys the natural flow of the phrase, which helps us to understand. When reading to the child, you can put a marker under the line of print being read so that he can follow along as you go. When the child wants to repeat what you have read, encourage him to read a phrase at a time, imitating your rhythm and intonation.

9. Avoid buying books that are your child's school readers. This is only likely to cause boredom without helping him to progress. Different books with equivalent language are much more likely to help him.

10. Reading should always be for pleasure or information and never become a task. We read because we enjoy doing so, or because we want to find something out.

11. Get the child to reconstruct a story from the pictures in a comic or book. This helps to teach the importance of sequence—not only of words in a sentence but also of ideas or events. Deaf children tend to be notably poor at this unless they have been carefully prepared for reading.

12. Relate reading to everyday life in a casual way. Road signs, shop signs, or frequently recurring captions on television programs can all be helpful.

13. Choose books that:

(a) are suitable to the age, ability, and interest of the child.

(b) have large print, are well spaced, and are written in natural phrases.

(c) have one or two sentences per page at first.

(d) have a controlled vocabulary with adequate but meaningful repetition.

(e) are very short and which can be read by the beginner at one sitting.

(f) are attractively illustrated for beginners. Books should have one picture for each idea or sentence.

(g) have pictures which stimulate verbal response from the child, preferably the actual words used in the text.

14. Encourage the child to engage in related activities that foster reading skills. These include:

(a) drawing, painting, and modeling—you can write a sentence or phrase to describe what the child has made, preferably using the child's own words.

(b) simple diary work. This forms a record of interesting events, with illustrations, which the child can help write and can then read and re-read. There is no need to write something for each day, as it would soon become tedious.

(c) the making of simple books by the child—about home, family, pets, etc. A page in such a book might contain a picture of his mother (drawn by himself) and under it the words "Here is Mommy."

(d) the tracing or copying of simple words, phrases, and sentences with accompanying drawing.

15. When looking at books with the child:

(a) be sure to discuss what the picture tells. Use simple questions.

(b) follow from left to right, top to bottom, beginning to end. (This is especially necessary with left-handed children.)

(c) discuss the main point first.

(d) ask the child to turn the page carefully.

(e) point out the numbers on the pages, if appropriate.

(f) ask the child the number of the page from time to time.

Basic Guidelines for Teacher/Clinicians

The following points summarize the main ideas expressed in this chapter as they concern teachers:

General

1. Follow an extensive pre-reading program such as we have outlined above before attempting to teach reading. Ensure that the child's auditory, visual, and spoken language skills have been adequately developed during the pre-reading stage.

2. When a child can recognize a few written words such as his name, "Mommy," "Daddy," and "airplane," you can teach him to read using a "look and say" approach. Use flash cards (either made or bought) to introduce the words that he will encounter in his first reading books. Teach him to read two or three new flash cards each day.

3. Make phrases or sentences from known flash cards before having the child read sentences in his first books.

4. Do not allow the child to look at your face as you read to him if he has any residual hearing. Make him follow what you read by looking at the book.

5. Ensure that the child hears the words that he reads and says them as clearly as possible so that he can make a correct mental association between heard, spoken, and written words.

6. Keep a record of the flash cards the child knows. Give him a star for each five new words he learns to read. Keep them on a chart so that he can see his own progress.

7. Remember that a child will initially find it easier to read words that are very different both to look at and to hear. Avoid the concurrent teaching of words which look or sound alike, e.g., *want* and *went*.

Writing

8. When writing, set a good example. Ensure that flash cards, wall charts, and transparencies provide excellent models for the child.

9. Make certain that the vocabulary of reading and writing are understood and can be used by the child. Such vocabulary includes words and phrases such as: "letter," "word," "sound," "big letters," "small letters," "that's too big," "leave a space," "begins with," "ends with," "first," "last," "beginning," "end," "same," "different," "right," "left," "up," "down," "straight," "another."

10. Have the child copy prepared sentence or word cards associated with pictures so that he becomes completely familiar with the shape of words being taught.

11. Be sure to use varied and appropriate materials such as large, unlined paper, books with only a few pages, a thick pencil or crayon, and blackboard and chalk.

12. Word cards should be prepared carefully. Print should be uniform and about the size which you expect the child to write in his book. Write the number of words on cards which the child will be able to write on the width of his page. He can then place the card exactly above his book and will be able to make a better attempt at copying. Copying from a blackboard is too demanding in the beginning stages.

13. Limit the initial choice of sentence forms to be read and copied. Be sure that pictures employed with them relate closely to the language used and that they are attractive, clean, and clear.

14. Spontaneous writing can be encouraged as soon as the children themselves indicate their desire to do so. This often happens as soon as they can read a few words. With very little encouragement, children will begin to write their own name and ask you to

show them how to write other words that interest them. When they draw a picture, they soon want to write something about it as they have seen you do about their paintings for wall display. Their writing gradually increases from a few words to a simple story. They enjoy reading each other's stories. They learn to refer to wall charts or very simple booklets made by you about "clothes," "games," etc. Later they can make simple dictionaries with words they can read. Spontaneous writing is fostered if the teacher/clinician writes brief stories to the child's dictation and shows the child how to use a typewriter—preferably with "jumbo type." The mechanical aspect of typing appeals to most children.

Phonics

15. Phonics should be introduced only when the child can already read at least 100 words. It is very important that the child should be able to say words plainly before he is introduced to the names and sounds of letters. He should be able to say "see," "so," "sat," for example, before he is told that "s" represents a certain sound. Otherwise he will make an association between a faulty sound and its symbol. The names and sounds can be introduced gradually, casually at first and when the child shows interest. When the child is ready, he will spontaneously remark on letter similarity. Writing lessons, which may take place about once a week, offer an opportunity to introduce the names of the letters casually. He can learn the alphabet and begin to do some spelling as soon as some letter names have been learned spontaneously.

Listening and Reading

16. Listening and reading can be jointly developed either by reading to the children or by having them listen to tape-recorded stories as they follow the text. Stories about everyday happenings, illustrated with sound effects, stimulate interest and provide the children with normal patterns of colloquial language. When dialogue is used, the child is supplied with expressions that he can employ in real-life situations.

17. Word or sentence cards can be used in auditory discrimination practice as well as in reading and writing exercises. The vocabulary can be chosen to suit the child's individual needs. Two or three cards can be placed on the table. The parent or teacher should read each card as she lays it down. The child should be asked to repeat each sentence. Then, the child is asked to look at

the sentences on the table and listen (without looking at the speaker). The child then points to the card which he thinks is appropriate and repeats the sentence. Practice of this sort leads to improved auditory skills.

Reference Books and Libraries

18. Simple dictionaries can first be made by the child. He can best learn the purpose of alphabetical order by being shown how to list the ever-increasing number of words he knows and requires for his daily work.

19. Reference books should be available in every classroom.

20. Workbooks aimed at extending language should contain interesting and factual material so that the child is building his general knowledge rather than doing meaningless exercises.

21. Materials available in the school, home, or library should be classified according to reading level so that the child can be sure of obtaining books that allow him to learn and, at the same time, enjoy the reading process at each stage of development. Only through the systematic organization of a hearing-impaired child's early reading experiences will he become able to read for pleasure and information throughout his entire life.

ANNOTATED BIBLIOGRAPHY

Clark, T. C.   Language and reading in the educational process of the hard of hearing child. In F. S. Berg and S. G. Fletcher (Eds.) *The Hard of Hearing Child.* New York: Grune and Stratton, 1970, pp. 331–348.

A brief but useful chapter on the subject of language and reading which should be read by regular teachers, teacher/clinicians, and parents.

Gibson, E. J., and Levin, H.   *The Psychology of Reading.* Cambridge, Mass.: The M.I.T. Press, 1975.

The authors are eminent psychologists deeply interested in perceptual learning and cognitive development. Although they approach the topic of reading from a standpoint of theoretically based research, the volume is very readable. Several topics touched on in this chapter are dealt with here in considerable depth, and graduate students and reading specialists will find it valuable. The book concludes with a section dealing with questions frequently asked about reading. One of these relates to "deaf" children and reveals the authors' restricted knowledge. The final word is reserved to acknowledge that parents can make a major contribution to their child's reading achievement.

Hart, B. O.   *Teaching Reading to Deaf Children.* The Lexington School for the Deaf Education Series, Book IV. Washington, D.C.: The A. G. Bell Association for the Deaf, revised edition, 1978.

Beatrice Hart supports our view that hearing-impaired children should have a good basis of spoken language before being taught to read. She describes how the preschool years can be used to advantage in preparing the child for reading instruction. Techniques and exercises for teaching reading at primary, intermediate, and advanced levels are provided. This book should be purchased by students, parents, and regular teachers, as well as by teacher/clinicians working with hearing-impaired children.

Huey, E. B.   *The Psychology and Pedagogy of Reading.* New York: Macmillan, 1908. Republished by the M.I.T. Press, Cambridge, Mass., 1968.

A delightful and fascinating account of the history of reading and writing, and of the various instructional methods used at the time of the book's original publication. Much of what was written then, remains valid today.

Kavanagh, J. F., and Mattingly, I. G. (Eds.)   *Language by Ear and by Eye: The Relationships between Speech and Reading.* Cambridge, Mass.: The M.I.T. Press, 1972.

This book is based on a research conference aimed at exploring the relationships between speech and learning to read. It will be of interest to those with a strong background in speech perception, linguistics, information processing and memory.

Russell, W. K., Quigley, S. P., and Power, D. J.   *Linguistics and Deaf Children.* Washington, D.C.: The A. G. Bell Association for the Deaf, 1976.

The authors conclude (p.206) that reading should be taught only after language has been developed through conversational interaction. They also provide important information for those preparing reading materials for hearing-impaired children. Parents would find some of the same information in more readable form in the January and February 1977 issues of *The Volta Review*. See also bibliography for the previous chapter.

Schonell, F. J., and Goodacre, E.   *The Psychology and Teaching of Reading*. Edinburgh, U. K.: Oliver and Boyd, 1945. Revised and republished, 1974.

This text, which was published under the senior author's name in 1945, has been supplemented and updated by the second author, who has retained much of the original text. North Americans may be unfamiliar with Fred J. Schonell, an Australian, and his pioneer work on the teaching of reading, spelling, and arithmetic and their remediation. This text is probably the single most practical book on the teaching of reading, and was written for parents as well as teachers. No elaborate theories are proposed. Although the book is written with normal-hearing children in mind, the topics dealt with—reading readiness, methods of beginning reading, the psychological factors involved, motivation of older children, etc.—are all equally applicable to hearing-impaired children. This soft-cover book should be purchased by teachers and parents working with hearing-impaired children. Available from the Longman Publishing Co., 55 Barber Greene Rd., Don Mills, Ontario M3C 2A1.

Schonell, F. J.   *Essentials of Teaching and Testing Spelling*. New York: Macmillan, 1954.

A systematic approach to the teaching of spelling to children aged 7 to 12. There are 3,200 everyday words which are intended to be studied in units of three to five words per day. Words are grouped according to similarity in auditory and visual elements, e.g., power, shower, tower; similar visual but contrasting auditory elements, e.g., stove, glove, prove; a combination of common elements and context, e.g., needle, thimble, button, cotton; common silent letter, e.g. knee, kneel, knock, knob. We recommend this approach to parents and teacher/clinicians working with hearing-impaired children.

Smith, F.   *Understanding Reading*. New York: Holt, Rinehart and Winston, 1971.

This book, subtitled "A Psycholinguistic Analysis of Reading and

Learning to Read," is mainly concerned about relationships between language and reading. It should be of interest to teacher/clinicians. The author has also written more recent books developing this theme further.

Stark, R. (Ed.)   *Sensory Capabilities of Hearing-Impaired Children.* Baltimore, Md.: University Park Press, 1974.

Essentially a report of a conference, this book includes an account of some interesting interchange on the topic of language and reading, including reading as a means of teaching language versus spoken language as a prerequisite for reading. A good index facilitates the location of relevant sections. Of interest to teacher/clinicians.

13. Program Designs for Individual Needs

A wide range of services is required in order to meet the individual needs of hearing-impaired children. In very few localities, however, is an adequate range of educational provision available. Services for hearing-impaired children are generally poor, due, perhaps, to the relatively small numbers of such children. It is easy for administrators to be apathetic about problems that affect only one in every thousand children unless considerable pressure for change is exerted by those directly concerned. It is hard for those concerned to exert such pressure unless they are informed about the services that could—and should—exist in any sizeable district. In this chapter we provide such information. We specify the components essential to a comprehensive system for the habilitation and education of hearing-impaired children, and indicate how the form and content of treatment can influence the development of verbal skills.

Population Variables

The Family

The fact that participation of parents (or guardians) is essential for successful habilitation, particularly in the first few years of life, has been stressed in previous chapters. It is sufficient here to emphasize that parental participation can be encouraged by the teacher/clinician and that the extent to which it occurs may be regarded as an indirect measure of the teacher/clinician's skills.

Parental aspirations also do much to determine the course of the child's development. If the parents wish their child to talk, and insist upon placement of their child in the form of program that

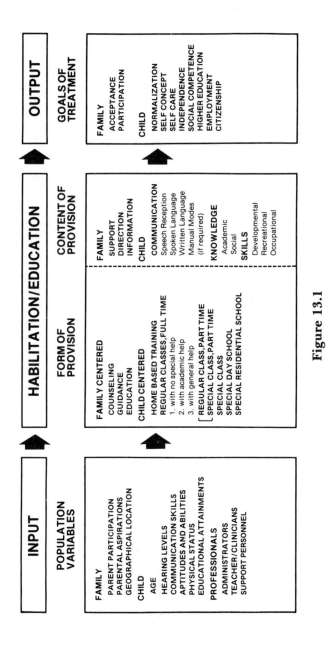

INPUT

POPULATION VARIABLES

FAMILY
PARENT PARTICIPATION
PARENTAL ASPIRATIONS
GEOGRAPHICAL LOCATION

CHILD
AGE
HEARING LEVELS
COMMUNICATION SKILLS
APTITUDES AND ABILITIES
PHYSICAL STATUS
EDUCATIONAL ATTAINMENTS

PROFESSIONALS
ADMINISTRATORS
TEACHER/CLINICIANS
SUPPORT PERSONNEL

HABILITATION/EDUCATION

FORM OF PROVISION

FAMILY CENTERED
COUNSELING
GUIDANCE
EDUCATION

CHILD CENTERED
HOME BASED TRAINING
REGULAR CLASSES, FULL TIME
1. with no special help
2. with academic help
3. with general help
REGULAR CLASS, PART TIME
SPECIAL CLASS, PART TIME
SPECIAL CLASS
SPECIAL DAY SCHOOL
SPECIAL RESIDENTIAL SCHOOL

CONTENT OF PROVISION

FAMILY
SUPPORT
DIRECTION
INFORMATION

CHILD
COMMUNICATION
Speech Reception
Spoken Language
Written Language
Manual Modes
(if required)

KNOWLEDGE
Academic
Social

SKILLS
Developmental
Recreational
Occupational

OUTPUT

GOALS OF TREATMENT

FAMILY
ACCEPTANCE
PARTICIPATION

CHILD
NORMALIZATION
SELF CONCEPT
SELF CARE
INDEPENDENCE
SOCIAL COMPETENCE
HIGHER EDUCATION
EMPLOYMENT
CITIZENSHIP

Figure 13.1

A comprehensive system of habilitation and education which has an input (a varied population), a range of treatment options (a variety of form and content), and an output (the achievement of certain goals). In this system, the treatment options and goals selected for a child depend largely upon the characteristics of his family, of the child himself, and of the professionals available to them.

encourages speech communication, then the likelihood is that, with their help, he will do so. In only a minority of cases are parents' aspirations for their child unreasonable. Parental aspirations can, of course, be modified positively or negatively through counseling, education, and experience.

The geographical location of the family can be an important factor both during the child's early years and throughout his schooling. Frequent, brief visits to a parent-infant center may be precluded when the family of a hearing-impaired child lives in a remote area. In such cases, intensive work for several days every few months may be substituted. During school years, the child may need to be placed in a foster home near appropriate day provision or attend a residential special school, unless the parent-infant program has equipped the parents and the child with sufficient skills that he can cope in regular class with little or no specialist help. Fortunate, indeed, are those families who live in close proximity to the type of program needed by the child, or can move to such a location.

The Child

The child's age affects choice of program in several ways. In the first few years there is no reasonable alternative to home-based training through the parents. If the parents are unable, for any reason, to function as the primary agents in the child's habilitation during the first three or four years, there is little or nothing that can be done to habilitate a child at that stage. From 3 or 4 years of age, the child can be taught directly by the teacher/clinician, but results will be limited unless there is parental collaboration that permits carry-over of treatment into out-of-school hours. The interaction of age with other variables also affects choice of placement. For example, a preschooler with limited spoken language skills can participate in virtually all of the activities in a regular nursery or kindergarten class, and such placement may be a vital adjunct to the special help he receives through parents and teacher/clinicians elsewhere. However, an older child with similarly restricted verbal communication could not be expected to share as fully in the classwork provided in a regular grade school. Similarly, academic achivement at a second-grade level might permit a 7-year-old hearing-impaired child to enter a mainstream class, but would prevent an 11-year-old from doing so.

Age at the onset of hearing impairment may be of considerable importance in determining the type of provision a child requires. If hearing impairment is present at birth, the child will tend to have a more restricted range of verbal experience than if he becomes hearing impaired after having heard his own voice for the first year or so of life, or if his hearing problem develops after he has acquired fluent, spoken language. However, the advantages of having heard speech and having acquired language can be quickly lost if the child is placed with nonverbal children (see Chapter 9).

Hearing levels are often treated as an index of expectation for the child: thus, if hearing impairment is mild, he is expected to achieve much; if it is profound, to achieve little. Standards of speech and academic achievement generally reflect this trend, but this indicates to us that a self-fulfilling prophecy is operating. To be sure, the greater the hearing impairment, the more difficult it is to learn and the slower initial progress may be. However, other things being equal, goals should be similar for both mildly and profoundly hearing-impaired children. The rate at which they acquire certain knowledge and skills may differ, as would the strategies selected to teach them.

Communication skills are the most significant variable in the selection of a program for the individual hearing-impaired child. Verbal ability is desirable to adequate performance in any setting, and mainstream education cannot be considered unless the child has adequate speech reception, speech production, and spoken language skills.

Aptitudes and abilities vary greatly from child to child. The greatest problem in placing a child according to these factors is that aptitudes and abilities are extremely hard to measure reliably. The most valid assessments are those that are undertaken by the skilled teacher/clinician in the course of her work. Flexibility in placement should be an integral feature of comprehensive provision. A child should not be kept in a setting which, in the course of ongoing diagnostic appraisal, is shown to be inappropriate for him. Such flexibility is particularly important in dealing effectively with hearing-impaired children who have other handicaps.

Physical status is generally a factor of about the same importance for hearing-impaired and normal-hearing children. However, when physical problems are so severe that they constitute an additional handicap, there is usually no alternative but to provide individual specialist help from a skilled teacher/clinician. This may be a temporary arrangement, as when the child is hospitalized for a spell, or a permanent form of provision. The special needs of hearing-impaired children, particularly the development of verbal communication, should not be delayed or ignored just because they also need treatment for physical defects.

Educational attainments may be expected to vary widely among students enrolled in special schools or classes, since their achievements are bound to reflect the extent and efficiency of earlier provision. Other things being equal, those starting late will tend to be far behind those who had parent-infant training. The attainments of hearing-impaired children who are enrolled in mainstream programs should be about equal to those of others in the class, although other members of the class may be a year or so younger. If the educational achievements of a hearing-impaired child do not match those of the majority of his classmates, either they or he will be adversely affected by such a placement. A hearing-impaired child does not always have to be average or above for him to be considered able to function with his hearing peers. For example, a slow-learning, hearing-impaired child may reasonably be integrated into a class of slow-learning, normal-hearing children.

The Professionals

There is a saying which goes, "If you are not part of the solution, then you're part of the problem." Administrators, teacher/clinicians, and support personnel who are well informed and working effectively toward a comprehensive system of provision are part of the solution. There are, however, far too many professionals who are part of the problem.

In general, educational administrators either appear to remain unaware of the possibilities that exist for hearing-impaired children, or they are not sufficiently challenged to act creatively. Few have taken the trouble to consider such children's needs in depth, or to initiate anything but token forms of care. Most are happy to accept propaganda that supports the simple, and demonstrably wrong, notion that one type of provision can meet the needs of all hearing-impaired children. Administrators are adaptable, however, and they respond positively to reasoned arguments, particularly if these arguments are backed by public pressure.

The teacher/clinician can successfully develop verbal skills in hearing-impaired children only if she has the necessary knowledge and skills to do so. A positive attitude toward speech communication is necessary but not sufficient for its achievement. Few teacher/clinicians currently have the required range of skills to foster verbal learning optimally among children with severe and profound hearing impairment. Those who do have such skills are the hearing-impaired child's greatest resource. Both the in-service and pre-service preparation of teacher/clinicians must be extended if the necessary range of knowledge and skills is to become commonly available. This will be discussed in the next chapter.

The concept that the assessment and treatment of a hearing-impaired child should be the concern of a team has been widely promulgated; but team effort has to be directed and coordinated. Our view is that the skilled teacher/clinician, the person who is to accept the main responsibility for the day-to-day management of the child, should be included on the team. Decisions on initial and subsequent educational placement should be reached by educators. There should be consultation with an administrator, an audiologist, a speech pathologist, a psychologist, and an otologist, and possibly with a pediatrician, a psychiatrist and a social worker. However, placement decisions should not be made by any one of these professionals. Direct educational management is not their specialty. Further, since adequate assessment of a child's aptitudes and problems can only be made in the course of ongoing treatment, the teacher/clinician and child should have continuing access to members of such a team. These professionals should be support personnel, in the truest sense of the term.

If the teacher/clinician has to function without access to support personnel, there is an obvious danger: She may fail to recognize certain of the child's needs or be unable to cope with them. There are equal dangers in working with a variety of professionals who do not function as a team: One professional may unduly emphasize the importance of a certain form of treatment, or parents and teacher/clinicians may receive conflicting information and advice. Few parents are in a position to resolve conflicting (or apparently conflicting) information, and most therefore react to that by doing little to help the child or to support the teacher/clinician. Alternatively the parents may consult other professionals, one after another. This course tends to lead to further confusion, frustration, and benign neglect of procedures that are essential to the child's habilitation.

Support personnel who are essential to effective programming also include technical staff whose work it is to ensure optimal function of hearing aids and classroom equipment and, in residential settings, personnel trained in child care. Teachers in regular schools may also be considered as support staff for children who are partially integrated into regular school activities, while teacher/clinicians may be regarded as support personnel for children who only need to receive occasional help when attending regular schools on a full-time basis. Support personnel should, of course, be consulted and involved as necessary while the child is enrolled in any program, and also when the child is being considered for placement in a different educational setting.

Form and Content of Provision

Special programs for hearing-impaired children can be either family-centered or child-centered. In the early years (0 to 3), there is no question that family-centered programs offer the most to a child, since no teacher/clinician can be as available or as emotionally close to the child as parents or caretakers. Learning at this stage takes place over relatively short periods of time, when the infant is alert, active, and receptive. Only by about 3 years of age has the average child developed enough capacity for sustained attention that direct professional intervention with the child becomes cost-efficient. Most child-centered training, i.e., training in which the professional works directly and consistently with the child, is begun about this age.

Family-Centered Programs

The form of provision that can be made in the early years of life may be considered as having three components: counseling, guidance, and education of parents. Direct work undertaken with the child in family-centered training is solely for the purpose of demonstrating strategies and techniques that the parents can use in the absence of professionals.

The content of counseling may be described as psychological support. It includes the reduction of parental anxiety, praise for the parents' achievements, and reassurance on matters relating to their feelings toward the child as a member of the family. Guidance includes providing the parents with directions for further work, how to evaluate the results of previous efforts, and what to anticipate as a result of further endeavor and interaction with the infant. The content of parent education will vary from family to family according to parental needs, interests, and abilities. Some parents are prepared to accept guidance without asking for detailed information as to why a particular course of action is being taken. Others would not find the content of this book sufficiently comprehensive, but would want to pursue information well beyond its scope. It matters little, providing that their efforts with the child are effective. Some of the parents with whom we have worked have never attempted to learn from books, yet through discussion and active participation they have done as much to develop verbal skills in their children as parents who were voracious readers. Support, guidance, and education can be provided for parents through group activities and workshops in which problems are discussed and shared.

Family-centered training can be undertaken in a clinic, a special room in a school, in a simulated home setting, in the child's own home, or in any combination of these. The more the teacher/clinician has to travel, the less time she will have available for work, the smaller her caseload will have to be, and the less cost-efficient her program will become. However, a certain number of home visits are an important adjunct to clinic- or school-based work, as they permit the teacher/clinician to make concrete suggestions relating to the use of materials and routines that are so much a part of the child's life. After all, the home is the actual environment in which most of his learning will take place. Suggestions relating to the installation of a loop induction system for the home, if this might be helpful, cannot be made without first seeing the size, shape, and relationships of the areas in which the child and his mother spend most of their time.

The teacher/clinician cannot work haphazardly in carrying out family-centered training. We have found it useful to plan in all three areas (counseling, guidance, and education) prior to every parent session, and to evaluate their session afterwards using the 12-point check list shown as Table 13.A.

As the child nears 3 to 4 years of age, the teacher/clinician can spend an increasing amount of time working directly with the child. We consider however, that the transfer from family-centered training to child-centered training should not be decided simply upon the basis of the child's age, but upon the relative contributions to his development that can be made by the parents at home as compared with those made by the teachers or teacher/

clinicians at school. Concurrently with effective parent guidance, children are able to attend regular nursery school for half-day sessions and thus extend their experience while at the same time allowing their mothers extra freedom. Such an arrangement can provide excellent data upon which to make decisions as to future placement.

TABLE 13.A

Parent Guidance: Session Check List

In this session, did you: —

1. know the child's present status in respect of
   (a) hearing and speech reception?
   (b) vocalization or speech?
   (c) comprehension of language?
   (d) communication?
   (e) educational or personal/social skills?

2. devise an adequate and sufficiently flexible session plan?

3. select material which was (a) interesting to the child?
                             (b) suited to his ability?

4. involve the parent(s) or family by: (a) discussing the child's progress and problems in communication and other skills and in general development? (b) having parents (family) take part in the session? (c) giving them direction (specific and general) and encouragement for the immediate future? (d) recommending sources of information or materials they might be seeking?

5. check and use the child's hearing aid and provide auditory experience?

6. put the child at ease and keep the child in a learning mood?

7. keep the child participating actively (even when you were talking to the parents)?

8. provide adequate reinforcement and feedback: i.e., make responses that were sufficiently differentiated for the child to learn from them?

9. encourage adequate vocalization and speech and successfully attempt to improve and extend vocalization and speech patterns?

10. check for comprehension at all times?

11. create and exploit numerous opportunities for the child to communicate throughout this session?

12. ensure that the parents went away from the session with a genuine sense of achievement and a clear understanding of various things they could do prior to the next session?

If you did not do all of these things, why not? Can you do better next time?

Child-Centered Programs

There has to be a wide variety of options open to hearing-impaired children if individual differences are to be catered to. Since parent-guidance work and associated intervention with the child under 3 years of age are carried out on an individual basis, differences among children in that age group are not determining factors in program selection. Differences among children, as discussed above, become important only when group treatment is begun.

The child's ability to communicate by speech is by far the most important of the variables that determine initial educational placement in a group. If the child can use spoken language effectively, then there is no major barrier to his placement in a regular nursery or kindergarten class. The majority of children born hearing-impaired who have received early treatment through an efficient parent guidance program, should be in this position. For them, the basic conditions of verbal learning will have been met, and there will have been the following:

1. early detection of hearing impairment,
2. early admission to a parent guidance program,
3. full-time use of residual audition,
4. guidance from a highly competent teacher/clinician,
5. parents who collaborated in the child's treatment program,
6. extensive exposure of the child to normal patterns of English,
7. adequate support services.

Unless they have only a mild degree of hearing impairment, children aged 3 to 4 years who have not had the advantages set forth above will not have acquired adequate verbal skills for regular class placement. Such children include those who have been in a poor quality parent-infant program and those who have had no previous training at all. The latter group will suffer, in addition to hearing impairment, the cumulative effects of sensory deprivation. Hence, they cannot be expected to learn spoken language at the onset of training as effectively as those who began treatment at an early point. However, experience with numerous cases indicates that a child can develop efficient verbal skills even up to age 9 or 10 if certain conditions are met. Even well beyond this age, improvement in verbal skills can be made if some training in spoken language has been provided during the early grades. The most essential conditions appear to be those specified as items 3 to 7 above. There may be other conditions, but they have not yet been clearly identified.

The burden of a handicap suffered by any child will increase with the number of the above conditions that are not, or cannot, be met. Thus if full-time use is not made of a child's residual hearing (item 3), he has to function as if his hearing impairment is more severe than is the case. His handicap will be increased, and his rate of learning will be less than optimal. If he makes good use of his residual hearing but does not have extensive exposure to normal English (item 6), an increased burden is imposed upon him. There are only so many additional burdens a hearing-impaired child can bear before progress in the acquisition of verbal skills becomes impossible for him. Reflection upon the forms of provision made for hearing-impaired children throughout North America and other countries suggests that few incorporate all of the conditions that enhance a child's opportunities for verbal learning. Most programs, in fact, are so structured that even excellent teachers are doomed to produce children with poor spoken language skills and low educational achievements.

It is easier for the necessary conditions for verbal learning to be met in some programs than in others. Thus a special class in the child's neighobrhood school, if staffed by a skilled teacher, can meet these conditions more readily than a residential special school. Residential schools can, of course, provide adequate opportunities for verbal learning, but not without considerable effort on the part of the parents, teachers, and the schools' administrators. Using the above conditions as a guideline, it is possible for parents who wish their children to have adequate opportunity to develop verbal skills to examine alternative forms of provision with the following general and specific questions in mind:

General
1. What are the aims and philosophies — avowed and practiced — of institutions?
2. What method of communication is used in teaching and in out-of-class activities (oral, manual, or total)?
3. What is the range of children admitted and criteria for admission: age, intelligence, degree of hearing impairment, aptitudes and attainments?
6. What are the limitations and advantages of the school's size (classification, individual attention, etc.)?
5. Are there adequate supplies of specialist equipment and other apparatus or materials?
6. Is the school amply staffed, and what are the teachers' qualifications? What is the pupil/teacher ratio?
7. What types of curriculum and syllabus are used and what are the general aspirations of the teachers?
8. What additional technical and other help is available?

9. What records are kept? Do these ensure continuity of each child's program?

10. Most schools have misfits (e.g., children with additional handicaps); what is the school's policy on these children?

11. What liaison does the school have with the parents, the community, hospitals, regular schools, employment agencies, consultants, etc.?

12. What is the general atmosphere (tone) of the program: is there a harmony of relationships and purpose?

Specific

1. Are both short- and long-term plans made for the class and for the individual child in all subject areas?

2. Do the teachers proceed from known to unknown; familiar to unfamiliar; simple to complex; easy to difficult? Are their materials suitable and well prepared?

3. Do all the children experience a sense of achievement while having the utmost demanded of them? Are they alert?

4. How does the teacher meet the requirements of the individual child while at the same time catering to all members of the class or group?

5. Is the teaching and the expected pace of learning related to individual variations in age, intelligence, hearing loss, and background?

6. Are the teachers creative in contriving and exploiting situations that promote speech and language development?

7. What types of reinforcement are provided?

8. What sort of relationships exist between the teacher and the children and among the children in the class? Do these relationships help or hinder learning?

9. Does the appearance of the rooms contribute to the children's education? Are they adequately stimulating and do they reflect the work and interests of the children?

10. How well do the teachers use special hearing aids, tape recorders, projectors, and other media? Do they pay adequate

attention to obtaining good signal/noise conditions? Are they able to recognize, locate, and remedy simple faults in hearing aids?

11. How well do the children use their hearing aids? Are all of them kept in prime condition? Are they worn in a suitable position? Is there a supply of hearing aids for loan in case of breakage? Do the children care for their aids within the limits of their ability and report faults which develop? What are the attitudes of both teacher and children toward individual hearing aids?

12. How often do the children have opportunity to interact with their normal-hearing peers?

The above questions can, of course, be asked in relation to any educational program and should be asked whenever transfer of the child from one program to another is envisaged. The questions cover both form and content of provision, and the answers that we would require to each are either self evident or covered elsewhere in this text. They should be considered in relation to the inherent advantages and disadvantages of the various forms of provision, discussed below:

Home-based training of children of school age is essential only for those who are not, for some reason, able to participate in classes of some kind. In such training, the teacher/clinician works individually and directly with the child. Children who may require such training include those who are not developmentally ready to learn through participation in group activities, e.g., severely retarded or otherwise multiply handicapped children. Children who suffer some long-term illness or disability may also require this form of help. The advantages of such a program are that they can involve parents maximally, and that all teaching is oriented to the specific needs of the individual child. Disadvantages include the possible isolation of the child from others, the difficulty of obtaining adequate support services, and the time consumed by the teacher/clinician. Only a small caseload of such children can be adequately served in home-based programs by one person, hence such programs are expensive to operate.

Regular classes can offer much to many hearing-impaired children, and a few children may be able to function adequately in such classes without additional support. Most, however, need some supplementary special help. Children who have a severe sensitivity gap usually require special types of hearing aids. Radio aids are usually helpful for them because they preserve the teacher's voice level over distance and provide a good speech-to-noise ratio (see Chapter 7). Children's progress in a regular class should be carefully monitored, and tutoring in both academic and speech communication skills should be provided as necessary.

Hearing-impaired children cannot be placed in regular classes and left to sink or swim. The class teacher must be adequately informed about the child's problems and be prepared to help meet the child's individual needs. Liaison of the specialist teacher/clinician with the regular class teacher is essential both prior to and during a child's enrollment in her class. Weekly contact with the teacher and child is essential to ensure his social adjustment and academic progress.

Parents, teachers, and administrators are often reluctant to place a hearing-impaired child in a regular class even when support personnel are available to the class teacher. There are sometimes good grounds for such reserve, since many regular class teachers have not been prepared by training to deal with handicapped children. However, children are not either handicapped or non-handicapped. There is a range of abilities and skills among both normal-hearing and hearing-impaired children. The mainstream of education is not made up of children who all function at average grade levels; there are fast and slow learners in every class. Some normal-hearing children may have more difficulty in learning new material than does a hearing-impaired child. Individual differences among normal-hearing children in a class may therefore be more diverse than between a mainstreamed hearing-impaired child and the normal-hearing counterpart who sits next to him. Nowadays, with current emphasis upon individual educational planning, the climate is more favorable toward mainstream education for hearing-impaired children than it has ever been before.

Only in a regular school can the range of experiences necessary to permit hearing-impaired children to function effectively in a world where 999 out of every 1000 can hear and speak be provided. The longer a hearing-impaired child gainfully attends a regular school, the better are his prospects of integrating fully into society at large. Given that mainstreaming is desirable at some point, what are the necessary conditions for admission to a regular class? Must the child be at average grade level for his age and able to communicate normally? Should the child be admitted to a special class or school only after he has demonstrated inability to cope in a regular class, or should he be placed in a regular class only when he has acquired certain arbitrarily determined levels of academic and communicative skills? The answers to these questions depend upon several factors.

There are no academic requirements for children of nursery school age, and children of this age do not need high-level communication skills in order to cope with nursery routines. At the outset they play in parallel, rather than in collaboration, with other children. Thus, most hearing-impaired children could function in a regular nursery setting. The extent to which they would benefit from such a setting could best be measured by how well the nursery activities fostered their verbal learning. Only if the teacher, the acoustic environment, the activities, and the other children in the nursery together promoted the development of a child's spoken language, would such placement be worthwhile. Such development could be optimally ensured by having a teacher/clinician available to supplement the work of the regular teacher. Under such an arrangement, most hearing-impaired children could begin their education in a mainstream setting. It would be economically feasible if the teacher/clinician were responsible for supplementary work with four or more infants, perhaps in different classes. No other form of provision could so adequately meet the conditions required for verbal learning.

The placement of hearing-impaired children in regular kindergarten classes, following nursery treatment as described above, could be organized in a similar fashion. At kindergarten level, there is little academic content, but great opportunity for the acquisition of spoken language. From background data on the child gained through such early mainstream placement, it could be determined whether regular or special provision would be required at grade school age. Admission to regular grade school classes is more complex because the child has to be able to cope with the academic content of the curriculum. A hearing-impaired child who has adequate speech communication skills but is a year or so behind in academic work certainly can be placed in a regular class at his grade level with slightly younger children; a large disparity in age between himself and his classmates, however, is to be avoided.

Most hearing-impaired children placed full-time in regular classes need to receive some form of special assistance. This is often most readily provided by an itinerant specialist teacher. Such a person can counsel the regular class teacher, discuss the child's current or anticipated problems with her, ensure that the child is making maximum use of residual hearing, monitor his progress in speech communication and academic skills, and provide remedial help as required. The task facing such a teacher is complex. It calls for flexibility and compromise in dealing with a wide range of teachers, children, and schedules. Children cannot be withdrawn haphazardly from their regular classwork. Traveling is time-consuming for the itinerant teacher, and careful planning is therefore essential to the efficient performance of her task. Mainstreamed children should, if possible, attend their neighborhood schools. This permits them to make social contact with children they will meet in out-of-school hours. However, where schools are widely dispersed, children may have to attend school in a more central location so that the itinerant teacher's travel time can be decreased and so that her caseload leads to a cost-efficient program of support. To place hearing-impaired children in mainstream settings without adequate support is to invite their failure. To provide such support to children who are correctly placed in regular classes largely ensures that they will continue to cope successfully with the demands of regular school life. The role of the itinerant teacher can therefore be considered crucial in a comprehensive system of educational provision.

Part-time regular/special class placement is probably the most economical and efficient means of bridging the gulf that usually exists between special and regular school provision. A special class in a regular school permits hearing-impaired children to receive part of their education from a specialist teacher and also share in regular school activities. They receive the help they need while they learn and grow in a normal social milieu. Most urban areas have sufficient numbers to support this form of provision, which can cater to children of diverse ages and abilities.

Several steps are essential in setting out to organize a special class in a regular school. First, one must select a school that caters to the age range of children for whom the special class is planned, a school in which the administrative and teaching staff are willing to be actively interested and supportive. The school selected must have sufficient numbers so that each of the hearing-impaired children can be absorbed into one class or another for different activities. Second, the classroom selected should occupy a quiet position in the school and be acoustically treated so that little noise is created by movement and so that reverberation is minimal. The room should be efficiently lighted so that speechreading is facilitated. Third, the room should be well equipped. Equipment should include one or more types of high-fidelity amplification systems (see Chapter 7), a tape recorder, an audiometer, the usual audio-visual teaching devices, and teaching supplies. Fourth, a highly skilled specialist teacher should be selected. In addition to her specialist qualifications, she should have a pleasing personality with ability to make and maintain good relationships with colleagues and parents. Since this form of work may isolate her from other specialist colleagues, she should be sufficiently self-reliant to function independently, and have the initiative to keep abreast of current thought and developments relating to special and regular educational treatment.

In most self-contained classes it is an advantage for the children to be fairly homogeneous in age and ability. This is not essential for a special class of six to eight children in a regular school. Indeed, diversity in age and ability among the children can be advantageous. Thus, while some of the younger or less able children are scheduled to participate in regular academic classes—or perhaps those that do not demand high levels of communication skills such as art, handwork, gym, games, etc., the older, or more advanced children can receive the undivided attention of the specialist teacher. Similarly, while the older, or more advanced children participate in academic work in regular classes, the specialist teacher can cater to the needs of the younger, or less able children. As the children treated become ready to integrate for more and more regular class lessons, so can new children be admitted for treatment. The teacher must have high-level skills to manage this type of work, particularly if she has limited access to support personnel who can help her in her task.

We have personally worked in all the areas of provision described in this chapter. Our experience has convinced us that work based on special classes in regular school offers more advantages and fewer disadvantages for school-aged hearing-impaired children than does any other form of program. Indeed, it was largely on account of our work some 20 years ago that special class provision became widespread throughout Great Britain. We were able to show that standards of achievement were generally better among children in special class/regular school settings and that the cost per child for this form of provision was about a quarter of that involved in residential school placement.

The efficiency of a special class in a regular school is not surprising in view of its advantages. We see these as follows:

1. It provides the greatest opportunities for hearing-impaired children to be in contact with normal-hearing adults and children. Hence their exposure to normal patterns of speech and behavior is maximized.

2. It permits the children to live at home as an integral part of the family unit and thus avoid the emotional trauma frequently engendered by separation from family.

3. Parents and siblings can receive continuing help and guidance from the specialist teacher at each successive stage of the child's development. This ensures that out-of-school hours are used to advantage.

4. Realistic adjustment to hearing impairment and the development of a good self image is facilitated by controlled contact with normal-hearing children at school and at home.

5. It provides opportunity for the child to take an increasing part in every aspect of regular school and community life, and to do so under the supervision of a specialist teacher over a period of years.

6. It avoids drastic change in lifestyle at the end of schooling. On leaving school, there are no radical adjustments for the child to make of the type demanded of children who have been living in a protected environment, segregated from hearing society.

7. The presence of a special class in a regular school in any locality helps to create public awareness of hearing impairment and the climate of opinion that most readily leads to the acceptance of hearing-impaired persons both in employment and social activities.

8. Teachers in special classes in regular schools remain in the mainstream of educational thought and endeavor. Working with regular class teachers and being in contact with normal-hearing children, they are constantly reminded of the normal

standards of communication and educational achievement for which they must strive.

To place several special classes rather than one in the same regular school leads to a severe reduction in the efficiency of treatment. This could mean that the opportunity for each child's individual participation in regular classes is reduced or eliminated simply because the regular class teachers cannot be expected to cope with several hearing-impaired children. Scheduling participation becomes too difficult. Thus, instead of extensive exposure to normal-hearing adults and children, regular classwork, and an abundance of normal speech and behavior patterns, the children receive treatment more typical of self-contained provision. The specialist teacher, unable to place her children in regular classes, has to teach larger groups, teach subjects such as art or physical education which do not require her special skills, and tends to be excluded from stimulating contact with the regular school staff and children. The loss of advantages in such a situation is too large a price to pay for administrative convenience.

The inherent weakness of a special class in a regular school is that its efficiency depends so much upon the quality of the specialist teacher and upon the collaboration of the school's nonspecialist staff. Opportunities for the hearing-impaired children to share in regular classes, in organized games and free play may be minimal unless the specialist teacher is alert to them. Parent participation may not be stimulated by a teacher who makes no efforts beyond the walls of her classroom or the hours of a school day. Similarly, the specialist with poor teaching skills will not systematically develop the child's speech communication skills and promote sufficiently rapid academic progress to enable the child to transfer full-time to a regular program. If such is the case, the special class will not serve as a dynamic bridge toward mainstream placement but as a static entity. (Of course, the results of poor teaching will restrict children's opportunity for growth in any form of program.) The advantages of being in contact with regular class teachers and normal-hearing children will also be lost to the specialist teacher who does not have the motivation to explore mainstream educational thought. It is unlikely that a specialist teacher who knows she has less than adequate skills or motivation will opt to work in a special class in a regular school. Work in such a class is far more open to scrutiny than in most other teaching situations, and weaknesses cannot be minimized through collaboration with other specialist staff.

Full-time special class placement may be essential for certain children for long periods, or the total duration, of school life. Such could be the case for certain mentally or physically handicapped hearing-impaired children. There are certainly good reasons for creating special classes in special schools for children who are unlikely ever to benefit from mainstream education. Thus a special school for retarded children might well need a special class for children who also have severe hearing problems. Conversely, a school for the deaf might need to create a special class for those who are retarded. We see no reason, however, why full-time placement in a special class housed in a regular school would ever be necessary. Even the most handicapped of hearing-impaired children can participate in some regular school activities.

Special day schools usually operate as part of the public school system of large cities or school districts. They can exist only where there are sufficiently large numbers of children who require full-time special education. There are substantial differences between a special day school and a special class attached to a regular school. For example, children in special day schools can be more closely graded according to their age and abilities. This permits them to be taught in groups. The teachers can be more readily supervised by the principal who, in most cases, is a more experienced specialist. Technical support services are easier to arrange. Teachers who specialize in certain subject matter can be employed. There is no doubt that these differences yield advantages for certain children. The inherent disadvantages of special day schools as compared with special classes in regular schools are that the children usually have to travel greater distances from home and have fewer opportunities to mix with normal-hearing children. To provide opportunities for hearing-impaired children to be taught with their hearing peers, some special day schools enroll a certain number of normal-hearing children in their classes, a process known as *reverse integration.*

Special residential schools are probably the most efficient solution to the problem of educating hearing-impaired children who live in remote or sparsely populated locations. Such schools may also serve hearing-impaired children from broken homes or economically disadvantaged families more effectively than any other form of provision. Large residential schools provide the opportunity for effective grading of pupils according to their age and abilities. However, they also tend to isolate them from normal-hearing adults and children, and thus reduce their opportunity for exposure to normal speech communication. Teachers and supervisory staff in residential special schools also tend to be isolated from society at large and from contact with those working in the mainstream of education.

There are a few private residential special schools that are structured so that their pupils learn sufficient academic and spoken language skills to transfer to regular high schools. Most public residential schools, however, tend to produce pupils who have poor academic skills and who sign rather than speak. Some of the lower standards found in public residential special schools may be attributed to the fact that, unlike their private counterparts, they have few selection factors operating in their favor. Few pupils of public residential schools ever acquire the skills necessary for transfer to regular schools. This being so, a high proportion of their pupils go on to special vocational training or to institutes of higher education that provide instruction through sign language.

Special Versus Regular Educational Settings

Throughout this chapter we have emphasized the advantages of mainstream education for those who can benefit from placement in a regular class. We are opposed to the provision of special education in self-contained classes or schools for any child who could, with reasonable support, benefit from a regular school education. However, mainstream education of hearing-impaired children cannot be successfully achieved without considerable effort. Parents must be consulted and involved in the decision making process. The staff of the school in which a hearing-impaired child is to be placed must be informed and accepting of the child's needs, and willing to meet them to the best of their ability. Specialist support for both the teacher and the child must be arranged. The regular teachers must be prepared to use special equipment such as radio hearing aids, if they are necessary, and to collaborate with the specialist in scheduling sessions during which extra help can be provided at times least disruptive to the child's participation in class activities. Regular evaluation of the outcome of mainstream work with each child must also be undertaken, and further individual work must be planned to meet whatever individual needs are thus demonstrated. Without such care, mainstream placement may have more disastrous educational and personal effects upon the child than would be created by special class or special school placement.

There are substantially more opportunities afforded for verbal learning in carefully structured mainstream programs than in most special education settings. There should, however, be no stigma attached to programs that are not in the mainstream of education or to the children who need to attend them. Every type of program described in this chapter is required. None can, or should attempt to, cater to the needs of all hearing-impaired children. Any program can be criticized if it unnecessarily restricts a particular child's opportunity for optimal verbal, academic, and personal-social development.

Goals of Treatment

Both the form and content of habilitation and education programs will be influenced by the goals set by administrators, teacher/clinicians, and parents. In this text we have emphasized the conditions required for the development of verbal learning. Different programs are not equally able to provide these conditions, nor are all their goals such that priority is given to spoken language skills. Placement of a child in a program should therefore be made only when the goals of the program, which help to determine the outcome of training, are made clear to the parents. Early family-centered work that provides parents with support, direction, and information is the most appropriate foundation for both parental acceptance of their hearing-impaired child and his needs, and family participation in the program selection process.

We favor programs that lead to normalization, that is, to the child's fullest possible participation in society at large. We recognize that hearing impairment is a handicap, but also stress that society is comprised of human beings with various levels of ability and types of aptitudes. To be normal, one does not have to conform with a statistical average in every respect or be like others in every way. To have particular weaknesses, strengths, tastes, and characteristics, and to be accepted by others in spite of them, is to be a normal individual.

The type of program in which a child is enrolled can do much to shape his concept of himself as an individual. If a child lives, learns, and grows in the company of normal-hearing children he will tend to identify himself as different from, but belonging to, normal-hearing society. Certainly it is better for a child to feel comfortable with himself as an accepted member of a "deaf" group than uncomfortable with himself as an unaccepted member of a "hearing" community. These are not, however, the only alternatives. Some hearing-impaired children can happily compete and conform with their hearing peers; some prefer not to be in the company of similarly hearing-impaired people; others like to have a foot in both camps. Self concept and adjustment are neither permanent nor absolute. Self concept can and should change with achievement and experience. Adjustment is relative to a situation. The goals of each program the child attends can nevertheless profoundly influence his development.

Self care can be fostered in any educational setting, but independence and social competence are certainly more likely to result from habilitation and education provided in a mainstream environment where the development of speech communication skills can best be encouraged. Ability to speak provides a greater potential for independence than signs, since speech is the universal means of communication. Unhampered by the need for an interpreter, a hearing-impaired person who can speak and understand speech is not so restricted in opportunities for social interaction as those who can only sign. Since hearing-impaired students who have good academic and speech communication skills can take regular college and university courses, many more subjects are open to them than to those who can only pursue higher education through special programs. Opportunities for prevocational training and employment are also more extensive for hearing-impaired persons who speak. Indeed, those who speak generally enjoy a high employment rate and good socio-economic standing. Well-educated, hearing-impaired citizens —whether they sign or speak—can contribute to rather than demand from society.

The purpose of any system is to produce. Study of the goals of present special education systems and the extent to which these goals are being achieved can only lead to a general dissatisfaction with current provision. Hopefully, the analysis undertaken in this chapter will suggest directions for effective change. However, new programs will succeed only if the personnel employed to implement them have adequate training and experience. It is to this topic—the training of professional personnel—that we turn in the next and final chapter.

ANNOTATED BIBLIOGRAPHY

Birch, J. W.   *Hearing-Impaired Pupils in the Mainstream.
Minnesota.* Leadership Training Institute/Special Education,
University of Minnesota. (Distributed by the Council for
Exceptional Children, 1920 Association Drive, Reston, Va.
22091.)
This is a report of a two-year study in which more than 200 people
involved in mainstream education of hearing-impaired children were
interviewed. In spite of the problems that are posed by mainstreaming,
the results of this study strongly and positively support the process and
use objective data to reject commonly ventilated armchair criticisms of
regular school placement. This inexpensive paperback is a must for all
administrators, teacher/clinicians, and parents concerned with
mainstreaming hearing-impaired children.

Brill, R. G.   *Education of the Deaf: Administrative and Professional
Developments.* Washington, D.C.: Gallaudet College Press, 1974.
This book was designed as a college text describing the development
of educational and rehabilitation programs serving the deaf in the
U.S.A. Particular emphasis is placed upon administrative and
supervisory aspects of special school work. This is essentially a brief
history of special school provision generously and fairly interpreted by
the author, a person who has contributed greatly to the advancement of
professional organizations, professional training, and the improvement
of special school provision in North America.

Cronbach, L. J., and Snow, R. E.   *Aptitudes and Instructional
Methods: A Handbook for Research on Interactions.* New York:
Irvington, 1977.
This is an advanced text on instructional theory that emphasizes
individual differences among children and the interaction between
aptitudes and the form of treatment children receive. It is by far the
most comprehensive discussion of individualized educational planning
available and is a must for all teacher/clinicians and administrators. It is
not written specifically with hearing-impaired children in mind, but
encompasses theories that are applicable to their treatment.

Elwood, P. C., Johnson, W. L., and Mandell, J. A. (Eds.)
Parent-Centered Programs for Young Hearing-Impaired Children.
Prince George's County Public Schools, 1977.
This book describes the various parent-centered programs for
hearing-impaired children in the State of Maryland. It includes
discussion of all the major facets of early intervention, beginning with a
description of some models upon which parent-infant work has been
based, identification procedures, diagnosis, audiological management,
organization of work and materials, multiply-involved children,
mainstreaming, and program evaluations. This text would be enjoyed
equally by parents, teacher/clinicians, and administrators. Ideas from far
and wide have been collected by the authors and editors and their
sources are clearly identified. References are also provided.

Nix, G. W. (Ed.)   *Mainstream Education for Hearing-Impaired
Children and Youth.* New York: Grune and Stratton, 1976.
A collection of essays, most by distinguished authors, all of whom have
been concerned with some aspect of educating hearing-impaired
children in regular schools in the U.S.A. Most chapters contain
references for further reading.

Northcott, W. H. (Ed.)   *The Hearing-Impaired Child in a Regular
Classroom.* Washington, D.C.: A.G. Bell Association for the Deaf,
1973.
This book was the first reasonably comprehensive treatment of
mainstreaming for hearing-impaired children to be published in the
U.S.A. Well planned and edited, it is full of interest and remains one of
the most informative texts about factors involved in regular class
placement: how to anticipate problems, recognize them, avoid them, or
deal with them in positive, creative ways. Numerous well-known authors
contributed chapters, most of which are well referenced.

Oyer, H. J. (Ed.)   *Communication for the Hearing Handicapped:
An International Perspective.* Baltimore, Md.: University Park
Press, 1976.
The services that are available for hearing-impaired people in 17
different countries are summarized in this book. Descriptions of the

form and content of various programs are provided in a way that such services around the world can be compared. References are given to studies that are quoted by the person(s) who wrote each chapter. All contributors are internationally known for their work with hearing-impaired children and adults.

Wilson, G. B., Ross, M., and Calvert, D. R.   An experimental study of the semantics of deafness. *The Volta Review,* 76, 408–414, 1974.

This is a brief article which examines the effect of labeling a child as "deaf," "hard of hearing," or "hearing impaired." It shows how the "self-fulfilling prophecy" operates—how the outcome of a child's education is influenced by the way professionals may initially classify his hearing impairment and needs. Their arguments are supported by experimental data and further references.

14. Preparation of Professional Personnel

*T*here is a serious mismatch between the range of services that are required by hearing-impaired children and the preparation of professional personnel who can provide these services. Programs for the preparation of teachers of the hearing impaired are almost exclusively geared toward the production of classroom teachers. To be sure, there is a need for specialist teachers who can work in self-contained classes, but there is also a need for professionals who can work competently in emerging services—in parent-infant programs, in special classes attached to regular schools, as itinerant teachers who can provide support for children enrolled full time in regular schools—and as supervisory personnel in special schools.

The generally poor standards of verbal and academic skills prevalent among hearing-impaired children, regardless of the type of program in which they are enrolled, indicate that the overall quality of current teaching is not consistent with present-day levels of knowledge in the field. Two questions must therefore be asked about the preparation of professional personnel. First, what kind of preparation is required for personnel who are needed to work in the emerging areas of service specified above? Second, what can be done to improve the adequacy of specialist teachers who work in self-contained classes? The two questions are closely related. Much of the knowledge and many of the skills required for successful work by each type of professional are common to both. Before attempting to answer these questions, let us examine the present situation in some detail.

293

Availability of Professional Workers

At present, the majority of teachers in North America who work with hearing-impaired children are not qualified to do so. Most have come to the field following preparation as regular teachers and have learned whatever special skills they may possess in the course of their work. The generally poor standards of verbal and academic achievements among hearing-impaired children can thus be attributed, at least in part, to widespread lack of specialist knowledge and skills. Many teachers who have received special training for work with hearing-impaired children fulfill only the provisional requirements for recognition (CED, 1972), namely successful completion of a one-year course involving 30 semester hours of preparation including practicum. Such limited preparation, at least prior to extensive experience, cannot fit a teacher to cope with the wide range of problems that are inherent in dealing with hearing-impaired children. While teachers with such training can carry out accepted educational procedures and may work effectively with children who pose no special problems, they cannot be expected to assume responsibility for parent-centered work, manage in unsupervised positions, or deal adequately with atypical hearing-impaired children unless they receive guidance from more highly trained and experienced personnel.

Knowledge relevant to the education of hearing-impaired children has grown substantially in recent years. Such knowledge, derived from advances in speech science, acoustics, auditory technology, audiology, psychology, phonetics, linguistics, and education cannot be acquired in the course of 30 or even 60 semester hours of training—training that must include abundant practicum. Few centers offer two-year specialist teacher preparation programs or cover material from the above fields in depth. It is therefore rare for currently available information—and the skills that can be derived from it—to be applied in the habilitation and education of hearing-impaired children. Can advances be promoted only by the preparation of more highly skilled specialists, or are there alternatives?

It has been suggested that the education of hearing-impaired children can be adequately covered by the collaborative efforts of three groups of professionals: teachers of hearing-impaired children (who would be concerned principally with academic instruction), audiologists, and speech pathologists. There is no evidence that such an arrangement can work or that it would be economically feasible. Indeed, there are several cogent arguments against such collaborative management of hearing-impaired children:

1. Parent-centered work with infants demands that one professional be recognized as the case manager. The potential for conflicting—or apparently conflicting—advice increases with the number of personnel involved. Parents faced with confounding advice can rarely become sufficiently committed to a course of action to work effectively with their child.

2. Small programs such as are necessary in areas with scant population—whether parent-centered or child-centered—cannot attract the number, variety, and quality of professional personnel that would be needed for day-to-day collaboration.

3. It would be uneconomical for several support specialists to be employed to help a teacher do what she could be reasonably expected to undertake if she were sufficiently skilled.

4. A child's progress is more likely to be fostered by a teacher/clinician who is capable of integrating knowledge and skills derived from several different professional areas than by a group of specialists with diverse skills. The skilled teacher/clinician would be less likely to unduly emphasize or neglect one aspect of the child's management relative to another.

5. Speech and hearing are not subjects to be taught, but basic elements in a communication system that is intrinsic to all educational activities.

There are, then, drawbacks in attempting to cover the direct habilitation needs of hearing-impaired children through the collaborative efforts of these three types of professional workers. However, there are greater obstacles to such collaboration in some areas of provision than in others. The greatest problems of a collaborative approach are to be seen in parent-infant work and in programs involving small numbers of children. In large programs which feature self-contained classes, collaborative coverage of a child's needs becomes administratively feasible. Such coverage is illustrated in Figure 14.1, which depicts how each of the three professions concerned—education of hearing-impaired children, audiology, and speech pathology—can be used to complement the others in providing aural habilitation and education.

Arrangements that are administratively feasible or expedient are not necessarily educationally sound. Thus, while it may be possible to utilize diverse professionals to cater to certain chil-

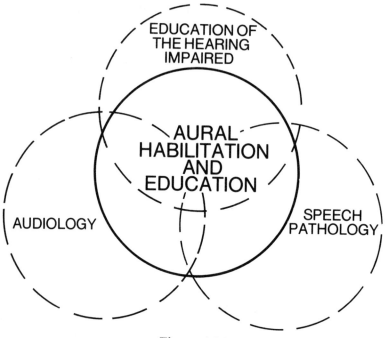

Figure 14.1

A diagram representing the areas of professional expertise (education of hearing-impaired children, audiology, and speech pathology) required for adequate coverage of aural habilitation and education services for hearing-impaired children. The merits of providing adequate services through the collaborative efforts of the three professional groups as compared with the employment of specialists who have the necessary training in all three areas to function relatively independently are discussed in the text.

dren's needs, it may not be desirable to do so. Teachers in self-contained classes would be able to provide better education for their children if they had many more of the skills possessed by audiologists and speech pathologists. This is not to suggest that class teachers should carry out audiological assessments and hearing aid evaluations, but to point out that better use could be made of hearing aids and children's residual hearing if such teachers knew when and why these procedures were necessary. Similarly, more high-quality, hour-by-hour spoken language instruction could be routinely carried out by teachers in self-contained classes if they had better speech science background than is generally the case. We see the specialist teacher as the person who must assume the responsibility for, and be able to integrate, all aspects of the child's special education. We do not consider that audiologists and speech pathologists should, in general, participate in direct teaching activities with school-aged children. They can, however, fill a vital supportive role with children enrolled in special classes or schools. We shall discuss the skills required by teachers in self-contained classes later in this chapter, following more extensive analysis of the nature of their tasks.

Personal attributes and experience, rather than professional labels, currently qualify persons for employment in parent-centered programs. There appears to be no strong reason for employing one rather than another of the three types of professionals for such work because, in general, none of them is adequately prepared for it through training. Parent-centered work calls for knowledge and skills in many areas, including infant development, parent counseling, differential diagnosis, acoustics, phonetics, audiologic assessment, hearing aid selection, hearing aid fitting, the use of residual hearing, the development of speech, language learning in normal-hearing and hearing-impaired children, and early childhood education. Typically, preparation for any of the three professions fails to encompass all of these areas. It does not include the several hundred hours of supervised practical experience with parents and infants that is essential if the professional is to integrate knowledge and skills from these diverse fields, utilize the information to the greatest advantage, and have well-founded confidence in her work.

People who have all of the skills required for work in parent-centered habilitation—those we describe in this text as teacher/clinicians—are rare. Most specialist teachers of hearing-impaired children have too little knowledge of speech science, audiology, and counseling; most audiologists have insufficient background in child development, speech science, language acquisition and education; and most speech pathologists have few, if any, skills relating to audiology, education, and the speech acquisition problems of hearing-impaired children. There is, therefore, a strong case for training personnel (teacher/clinicians) specifically for work in parent-infant programs. Such training should be extensive.

There is an equally strong case for requiring more extensive training for teachers who are destined to manage a special class in a regular school or to provide itinerant support services for children enrolled in regular classes. Such teachers have to be relatively independent of other professionals in much of their work. Certainly they need access to support personnel but, in most situations, they cannot expect to have day-to-day assistance from an audiologist, speech pathologist, or technician. Higher level training is also essential for those who intend to assume supervisory positions in special schools.

Types of Personnel Required

Specialist teachers and teacher/clinicians are faced with a variety of tasks in the habilitation and education of hearing-impaired children. Do all of these tasks require diverse, high-level knowledge and skills? How far is it possible to delegate some of them to assistants with less extensive professional training? These questions are among the most important that can be asked in relation to the preparation of specialists, for they are basic to the feasibility, cost, and efficiency of any program. It would be highly uneconomical for a person who has diverse, high-level abilities to be employed in a situation that demands their use for only a small proportion of her time. An analysis of the tasks involved leads us to suggest that personnel with various levels of preparation can, and should, be involved in all types of programs, but that higher level skills are generally required in those aspects that bear upon verbal learning.

Decision and Delegation

A person with diverse, high-level skills must be responsible for decisions affecting the course of each child's treatment. The decisions the teacher/clinician makes are often difficult. They may have to be reached in the face of rapidly changing circumstances, uncertain predictions about the results of a course of action, reactions that are difficult to observe, ambiguity underlying the child's responses or failure to respond, and the availability of support staff. Her decisions, which must be made in relation to the needs of the child as a whole as she perceives them, may critically affect the child's short- and long-term progress. The extent to which she can safely delegate work with the child to others will depend upon the confidence with which she can make decisions. Let us illustrate and discuss the bases of decision making.

Changing circumstances are most commonly encountered as a result of a shift in parental attitudes, maturation of the child, the results of treatment, or all three factors. In very young children, such changes can be both substantial and rapid. Thus, in parent-infant work with children aged 0 to 4 years, the specialist must be able to respond speedily to new requirements if she is to foster optimal progress. In older, school-aged children, change is much more gradual. The relative stability of circumstances in school-based work renders it possible for treatment specified by a highly trained teacher/clinician to be carried out by an assistant with less (but sufficient) knowledge and skill.

The uncertainty of prediction as to the outcome of habilitative measures is a problem that plagues teacher/clinicians. The predictability of results is, of course, always better for short- than for long-term treatment. Predictions as to the outcome of training can only be made on the basis of thorough familiarity with the child: his problems, his aptitudes and abilities, and his past performance. Prediction is, therefore, more likely to be accurate with older than with younger children because better estimates of performance can be derived from past experience with them. Thus, the use of less skilled assistants may be feasible in child-centered, but not in parent-centered, programs.

Reactions that are difficult to observe are common among hearing-impaired children of all ages. The most difficult of reactions to observe are those relating to verbal communication and its development. One cannot easily determine how much a child has detected, discriminated, identified, or comprehended of a spoken utterance. Indeed, a child may understand a message completely, yet not react overtly to it. Alternatively, evidence that a child has heard and understood what was said may not be immediately forthcoming: there may be a considerable delay before the child responds. The child may be able to understand vocabulary that he does not use, or use vocabulary that he does not fully understand. The meaning that the listener derives from what the child says may not be what he intended. The child's ability to produce a particular sound may not be evident from his use of spontaneous speech. Verbal communication is of primary importance in the habilitation and education of hearing-impaired children. All specialist workers engaged in parent-centered or child-centered work must therefore be able to elicit, interpret, and base further work upon reactions that, for the layman, are difficult to observe. Without such skills they cannot be considered as competent specialists.

Ambiguities underlying the child's responses or his failure to respond call for considerable interpretive skill on the part of the teacher/ clinician. Several possible interpretations of responses can be missed by a professional who does not have adequate training. Thus a child may respond as requested when asked to bring a shoe because he has deduced from the prevailing situation that a shoe is required; not because he has understood the verbal request. Teachers who are not thoroughly aware of possible ambiguity in any such response have insufficient skills to determine a child's level of language comprehension with accuracy. Therefore they cannot guide his language development effectively. Highly skilled teachers are not satisfied simply with obtaining a desired result: They constantly seek to determine what factors in their work, or in the child's experience, led to that result.

Hearing-impaired children frequently confuse one spoken message with another. Thus, in answer to the question, "How old are you?", they might reply, "Very well, thank you!" In such a case there is ambiguity as to the cause of the child's misunderstanding. The skilled teacher/clinician will not just clarify the question for the child, but will seek to determine why an inappropriate response was obtained and to remedy the problem. In this instance, the likely cause of the inappropriate response would be visual confusion of the two common questions, "How are you?" and "How old are you?" Such errors point to the need to ascertain why the child did not hear that there were four syllables in the question, not three. Was the child's failure to hear the difference due to his hearing impairment, a faulty hearing aid, or to temporary or habitual lack of attention to auditory patterns? Effective action to remedy the problem would depend on an accurate diagnosis of its cause. Such diagnosis would be beyond the capability of a teacher who did not have high-level knowledge and skills in education, acoustic phonetics, speech perception, and audiology. The highly skilled teacher/clinician would not have to consult other specialists about such a problem because her knowledge of these different fields would be adequate and integrated.

Ambiguities relating to the speech production capabilities of hearing-impaired children are very common, and only a highly skilled person can resolve them. There are several reasons why a child may, for example, substitute [b] for [m], be unable to produce a particular sound pattern, develop faults such as nasalization, neutralization, or prolongation, or fail to use sounds in meaningful speech when he has the capability to do so. A teacher who is unaware of the many possible reasons for inadequate speech production cannot diagnose the child's problems. In her hands, the best that the child can do is enter a holding pattern — continue to approximate speech patterns as best he can. With prolonged practice, faulty approximations become habitual and resistant to change even under the guidance of an exceptionally able speech teacher.

There can also be considerable ambiguity underlying a child's lack of response to a stimulus, for there are many reasons why a child can perceive something, yet not react to it. It takes considerable expertise to structure situations for young children so that they are almost certain to respond when a stimulus is presented. With older children, the task is less difficult. Nevertheless, there must always be skilled exploration of the possible reasons when no response is obtained from a child. If there is not, serious mistakes that render both diagnosis and treatment invalid can be made.

The availability of support staff is, of course, a prerequisite for the delegation of specific tasks. If nobody is available to assume responsibility for certain aspects of work, then the teacher/clinician must decide whether she can undertake them herself or whether the child cannot be given the assistance that he needs. In parent-centered work, the teacher/clinician's task is to help the parents carry out the habilitative work with the child. She may delegate the child's auditory assessment to an audiologist, but would be wise to control the selection and fitting of the child's hearing aids herself, since the validity and reliability of the procedures involved depend upon ongoing evaluation in the course of the child's training. Delegation of hearing aid repairs to a technician should, of course, be an accepted policy. Decisions relating to the need for help from another professional, such as an otologist, a psychiatrist, or a social worker should be made in consultation with the parents. We are convinced that parent-centered work cannot be successfully delegated to a professional who does not have the range of high-level skills discussed above.

Teacher/clinicians who deal with hearing-impaired children in regular schools — whether or not the children are enrolled part-time in a special class — function in a system in which some of their pupils' habilitation and education are routinely delegated to others. Their task is to decide which, and how many of the child's needs, they themselves should cater to. Their decision will vary

according to the characteristics of the children, the type and quality of regular school provision, and the location of the child or
special class. In remote areas, there may be few, if any, ancillary
services close at hand and hence no opportunity to delegate tasks
to support personnel.

Highly skilled specialist teachers in special schools are in the
most advantageous position to supervise whatever work they delegate to others. Thus, if staff with skills of the type that can be
acquired in one-year training programs are to be employed, they
could serve most usefully in special school programs for hearing-
impaired children.

The critical nature of decisions made by professionals concerned with
hearing-impaired children cannot be overemphasized. Decisions
based on accurate assessment are crucial to the adequate selection
and fitting of hearing aids, without which habilitation and education cannot be optimally effective. Inappropriate decisions relative to early intervention can permanently and adversely affect a
child's development. Decisions leading to the placement of a child
in a regular or special program can have enduring consequences
on the child's ultimate achievements and his future role in society.
Within such programs, day-to-day decisions can also have lasting
effects. An inappropriate decision relative to a young child can
destroy the parents' confidence in the person who is providing
counseling and render them unable to work happily and effectively as the prime agents of habilitation. The teacher's apparently
trivial decision to seat children in a particular manner in class can
place pupils outside the range over which they can hear her voice
and therefore slow their progress. Her decision to teach speech in
a particular manner may lead to faults that are difficult or impossible to eradicate at a later stage. Her decision to use a highly
structured rather than a guided interactional approach in teaching language may result in restricted or stereotyped linguistic
function. Her decision to teach mainly through group instruction
may prevent individual children from making optimal progress or
even to lose skills acquired through previous training.

The enormous number of critical decisions that have to be
made leads us to suggest that it is generally unsafe and harmful
for the development of hearing-impaired children to be supervised by anyone other than highly trained professionals. The potential for disservice to be rendered by an inadequately qualified
person increases in proportion to the degree of hearing impair-

ment suffered by the child. Thus, although there is more scope for supervision of staff in a special school, if that school caters mainly to the more severely hearing-impaired children, delegation to less well qualified staff may result in ineffective treatment. The effectiveness of teaching by less skilled staff will depend on the characteristics of the children and the amount of supervision that can be provided.

Levels of Training

Our task analysis (above) indicates that the majority of personnel engaged in the habilitation and education of hearing-impaired children should have more diverse knowledge and higher level skills than is presently the case. We are engaged in the preparation of specialist teacher/clinicians and find that even carefully selected personnel, who are already qualified teachers, require not less than two years (60 semester hours) of specialist preparation and integrated practicum in order to deal effectively and relatively independently with the varied and complex problems met in direct work with hearing-impaired children. Further training and/or experience could reasonably be demanded of those who wish to teach multiply handicapped hearing-impaired children, assume positions in special school administration, work in teacher preparation programs, or do research. Less training might be required of those who wish to work as assistant teachers and less again for those who are prepared to function as teachers' aides. The following four types of personnel are thus delineated:

Level 4: The Leadership Person would be concerned with the critical assessment of theory or practice, would design and supervise treatment programs, direct research, evaluate treatment procedures, train teachers and teacher/clinicians, undertake administration, contribute books and articles to the literature, promote the functions of professional organizations, and be able to describe both broad and detailed aspects of the field to agencies, other professionals, and to the public. Usually this person would have at least five years of professional preparation plus experience and hold a Ph.D. degree.

Level 3: The Skilled Teacher/Clinician would be concerned with the supervision of other teaching personnel, would collaborate with those in related disciplines, interpret data generated by other professionals, apply highly specialized testing and remedial procedures, identify factors influencing the effectiveness of treatment, specify possible causes for ambiguity in responses or reasons for failure to respond, establish priorities in teaching, prescribe programs for atypical hearing-impaired children, be directly involved in parent-centered programs, manage a special class in a regular school, and/or provide counseling for parents of children at each stage of their development. Usually the teacher/clinician would have at least two years of specialist preparation following training as a regular teacher, or have equivalent training and experience, and hold a master's degree.

Level 2: The Specialist Teacher would normally be employed in a special school but could, given sufficient experience and/or supervision, assume responsibility for a special class in a regular school or itinerant teaching work. The specialist teacher should be able to apply a wide range of special procedures to elicit various desired behaviors, interpret complex responses (some of which might be difficult to discern), safely and effectively carry out routine educational procedures, follow prescribed procedure for helping atypical hearing-impaired children, and recognize the need for assistance in, and seek to remedy, areas of professional weakness. (At present the main areas of weakness among specialist teachers are those relating to the development of their pupils' verbal abilities and spoken language skills.) Usually the specialist teacher would hold a bachelor's degree in the education of hearing-impaired children, or a bachelor's degree and a postgraduate diploma or master's degree in the education of hearing-impaired children. Most post-graduate diplomas and master's degrees in this area are awarded following a one-year (30 semester hours) period of preparation.

Level 1: The Teacher Aide would usually be employed in a special class to carry out routine tasks that call for little or no interpretation of the child's responses. Such aides can free the specialist teacher or the teacher/clinician so that she can undertake work that requires her knowledge and skills. With on-the-job training and supervision, an aide can acquire many special skills and assume an increasingly important role in the teaching process. Indeed, in successful parent-centered programs, the parents initially function as the teacher/clinician's aides and then become the primary agents in their child's habilitation. No formal pretraining is necessarily demanded for employment as a teacher aide, although certain personality, educational, and social characteristics are prerequisites for this type of employment.

Personnel at each of the above levels have to do more than promote children's progress in communication skills, academic achievements, and social competence. They must also contribute to each child's well being as an individual: They must respect his dignity, enhance his self confidence, minimize his anxieties, prevent boredom, help him develop human values, and generally encourage him to feel that both he and life are worthwhile. They must also have a positive attitude to their work, one which pervades their activities with the children.

Professional Knowledge and Skills

There have been many attempts to define and classify the knowledge and skills required by specialist teachers of hearing-impaired children. Basically, the impetus for this work stemmed from the need to specify the form and content of teacher preparation programs. Without a list of competencies that had to be acquired by students aspiring to enter the field, both those engaged in teacher preparation and those responsible for its funding were working without guidelines. They were also without a yardstick for measuring the results of their efforts. The lists of competencies published to date have spawned a small number of research studies. Most were designed to determine which competencies teachers considered to be most important. These studies have also generated ideas and opinions which have received widespread discussion. The current trend in teacher preparation programs across North America is toward competency-based training, that is, teaching students why and how to perform specific tasks. This trend accords with educators' general acceptance of the desirability of setting behavioral objectives—clearly defined goals for teaching. The trend is also supported by administrators since, when questions of accountability for expenditures of public funds are raised, they can point to the acquisition of specific competencies among trainees as concrete evidence of a program's worth.

The Definition of Competencies

Actually, the competencies listed in various publications relating to the knowledge and skills required by teachers of hearing-impaired children are neither objective, concrete, nor specific. Most have been derived through the process of introspection on the part of specialist teachers. This is not to say that they have no validity, but to stress that they have, by and large, been subjectively determined. That competencies as currently delineated are neither concrete nor specific is best illustrated by the following items drawn from lists presently in circulation: "The teacher should be able to recognize the physical, acoustic and visual characteristics of the learning milieu conducive to meeting the needs of the hearing-impaired learner and to appraise the educational setting in school, home and community"; "to recognize the individual differences of each deaf pupil and to make provision for these"; "to demonstrate confidence and competence in relating to other professionals, parents, and infants"; and "to implement appropriate instructional procedures."

There may be no feasible alternative to broad, subjective definition of the competencies required of the four types of personnel described earlier. Objective definition of the knowledge and skills that have to be acquired in order to work effectively in each type of program described in the previous chapter would be possible only if someone other than the specialist could specify the nature of the work she does. Successful specialist personnel—those whose work usually leads to the satisfactory achievement of the program's goals—could be located and observed, but it is doubtful whether the thousands of interactions observers would see between the professional and the child (and/or his parents) could be adequately recorded, interpreted, and classified. The presence of the observers would influence the professional's work; even if the observers were able to record the events that occurred, it is doubtful whether they could clearly determine their significance or specify the types and levels of knowledge and skills underlying them. If the observers were, themselves, more highly skilled than the professional they were observing, they could make judgments (albeit subjective) relative to these things. Such judgments of highly skilled observers are, of course, widely accepted, for all students training for the field are observed by their supervisors and pass or fail their practicum on the basis of such judgments.

Attempts to be specific in the definition of required competencies can lead to many problems. Given that all of the broad areas of knowledge and skill needed by the specialist could be agreed upon, how much detail should be contained in the definition of a competency? To define the knowledge and skills embodied in a competency in broad terms is to be vague; to define them in detail is to be specific, but perhaps trivial. Furthermore, detailed definition of required competencies would lead to the generation of lists containing many thousands of items and would obscure important inter-relationships between certain areas of knowledge and skill. Let us use speech teaching as an example to illustrate these points.

Ability to teach speech production skills is an important aspect of habilitation and education of hearing-impaired children. It is, however, too large an aspect to be satisfactorily regarded as a single competency. Speech acquisition may be considered as a process that consists of several distinct stages of development, with many target behaviors to be mastered in each stage, and with a variety of subskills underlying each target. The knowledge required to foster speech acquisition effectively stems from several areas, including acoustics, phonetics, linguistics, anatomy, physiology, and psychology. We cannot find a satisfactory way to specify the range of competencies required for this single aspect of habilitation. One cannot meaningfully list a series of competencies based on each stage of acquisition because speech behaviors acquired by the child at one stage also occur in subsequent stages: they are not distinct. Similarly, one cannot specify competencies relating to each target behavior because many mechanisms, possible faults, teaching strategies, and areas of knowledge are common to several of them. One cannot economically specify competencies relating to each subskill because there are thousands of them. Beyond this, the professional is not just teaching speech, but teaching speech to hearing-impaired children who differ in age, hearing levels, aptitudes, and abilities. There is no simply defined competency that can describe the variety of ways in which the professional has to be able to develop a given stage, target behavior, or subskill of speech so that such development is related to the needs and characteristics of each individual child as a whole, dynamic being.

In summary, there are evident weaknesses in the notion of competency-based professional training. It may not be possible to define meaningful competencies in all required areas of knowledge and skill. When such definition is possible, the competencies defined will be based on subjective opinion. Lists of competencies will tend to reflect the experience of senior professionals who may not have experience in current emerging services or advances in related fields, with the result that competency-based training may operate to preserve the *status quo*. It may prevent students from receiving satisfactory training relating to emerging services, new ideas, and technological developments. Competency-based training founded on inadequately formulated lists may also lead to concentration upon the training of certain areas of knowledge and skills while detracting from the importance of their inter-relationships. It could lead to an emphasis on methods rather than principles, and hence to a rigidity of thought and practice among a program's graduates. If such weaknesses are not avoided, personnel will be produced who can neither think, plan, nor teach creatively.

There is, however, need to specify the required content and standards of preparation programs in terms that are as concrete as possible. Weaknesses in the process are most likely to be avoided if university staff, administrators, and professional personnel work jointly to define the knowledge and skills essential to their particular form of provision. Such collaboration must also extend into the theoretical and practical preparation of personnel. Students in training must be given opportunity to hear about, observe, and participate extensively in the work carried out by successful professionals.

The Logistics of Preparation and Staffing

More highly skilled personnel (Level 3 and Level 4) are required if effective, comprehensive systems of habilitation and education are to be provided. Without such professionals, adequate parent-centered work cannot be offered, special classes attached to regular schools cannot be properly staffed, sufficient itinerant support specialists cannot be provided, and ongoing supervision and in-service training of teachers in special schools cannot be improved. The supply of teacher/clinicians can only be ensured if parents, teachers, and educational administrators recognize the need for them, and if more training programs become oriented toward their preparation.

There are several ways in which more highly skilled teaching personnel can be prepared. First, they can be required to experience more extensive preservice training—training that cannot occupy less than two years. Programs for the preparation of audiologists, speech pathologists, and teachers of hearing-impaired children could gear themselves toward producing this "new breed" of professional, the Level 3 teacher/clinician who has the necessary skills in all three areas of expertise. Second, personnel who are already qualified as members of one of the three professional groups could be trained in areas of weakness. For example, specialist teachers of hearing-impaired children (Level 2 personnel) could return to graduate school for further training in various aspects of audiology and speech and language pathology. In such programs the purpose would be not merely to cover the content material, but to help the students integrate knowledge from all three areas through seminars and practicum experience. Third, skills of specialist teachers in self-contained classes can be increased through in-service training and by short-course attendance. We are currently providing all three types of preparation and find that each has its advantages. Most difficult is the in-service training of personnel, since essential knowledge of other areas cannot be readily gained by teachers who are occupied with day-to-day planning and management of special classes. The most appropriate way to help improve standards, it seems, is to ensure that specialist teachers have constant access to teacher/clinicians on staff who can serve as consultants and supervisors.

There is need for personnel with particularly high-level skills to work with children who have handicap(s) in addition to hearing impairment. To date, special training to meet the needs of such children has been very difficult to obtain. If education rather than custodial care is to be provided for many such children, teacher/clinicians with considerably more expertise must be trained and become available.

The cost of training and employing more highly skilled (Level 3) personnel is clearly greater than that involved in the preparation and engagement of specialist (Level 2) teachers. However, cost cannot be considered as an isolated factor. If a teacher/clinician can do certain work that a specialist teacher cannot, or if she can work more efficiently than a specialist teacher, actual costs per pupil can be reduced.

We are convinced that excellence in the verbal performance of most hearing-impaired children is a realistic goal. However, verbal learning can be efficiently fostered only if more highly qualified personnel are prepared and utilized within all the types of programs encompassed by a comprehensive framework of habilitation and education. Those concerned with hearing-impaired children must decide to either accept the mediocrity of present programs or to accept the challenge to work for the improvement of provision through the use of more extensively trained personnel. Their choice, in the long run, will determine whether or not opportunities for verbal learning, spoken language skills, and reasonable academic achievements will be open to most hearing-impaired children.

ANNOTATED BIBLIOGRAPHY

Council on Education of the Deaf.   *Standards for the Certification of Teachers of the Hearing Impaired.* Washington, D.C.: The A. G. Bell Association for the Deaf, 1972.
This booklet broadly defines the type and standards of preparation required for CED certification as a teacher of hearing-impaired children. It specifies the required content of training for provisional certification (a minimum of 30 semester hours) and professional certification (3 years teaching experience plus 20 semester hours of advanced study beyond provisional certification). It also lists the major competencies required of specialist teachers of hearing-impaired children.

Hehir, R. G.   Competence based teacher education for teachers of the deaf: the issues from the state level. *The Volta Review,* 77, 105–116, 1975.
This article describes the requirements for specialist teacher certification in New York State, and how competencies demanded of teachers of hearing-impaired children are defined by consortia consisting of university staff, administrators, and professionals working in collaboration. The need for differential training for teachers at various levels and in alternative educational settings is stressed.

Northcott, W. H.   Competencies needed by teachers of hearing-impaired infants, birth to three years, and their parents. *The Volta Review,* 75, 532–544, 1973.
This article describes a study of the competencies required by personnel involved in work with hearing-impaired infants and their parents. The study follows the format of those published by the U.S. Office of Education (see below). References to relevant work are provided.

U.S. Office of Education. *Teachers of Children Who Are Deaf.* Bulletin No. 6. Washington, D.C.: Department of Health, Education and Welfare, 1956.

This document reports the first major attempt to specify the competencies required of specialist teachers of hearing-impaired children, and to have these competencies rated in importance by classroom teachers. Ability to teach language and speech were ranked more important than all other competencies, but teachers considered themselves ill-prepared for these tasks.

U.S. Office of Education. *Teachers of Children Who Are Hard of Hearing.* Bulletin No. 24. Washington, D.C.: Department of Health, Education and Welfare, 1959.

This document is similar in most respects to Bulletin No. 6 described above. Teachers' rank ordering of the various competencies indicated that most considered abilities relating to the teaching of speechreading to be of the greatest importance. In modern work, which gives greater emphasis to the use of residual hearing, competencies would surely be ranked very differently.

Index of Authors

Index of Subjects

A

Acoustic properties of speech, 65–75
 and hearing impairment, 74
Acoustics
 and auditory sensitivity, 120–122
 of the teaching environment, 121, 283
Administrators and education provision, 15–20, 270–272
Age of child
 and acquisition of verbal skills, 276
 and brain plasticity, 195
 and control of speech mechanisms, 181, 185
 as an educational variable, 268–269
 and language milestones, 32
 and onset of hearing loss, 29–30
 and part-time special class placement, 283
Aided audiograms, 118–119
Air conduction of sound, 62–64
Alphabet, the, 247, 249
Ambiguities
 in child's responses, 79, 300–301
 in speechreading, 135–138
Amplification
 binaural-monaural, 103–105
 parameters of, 88–90
 provision of, by parents, 12
 see also Hearing aids
Aptitudes
 as a factor in educational placement, 269

Assessment
 see Evaluation
Audiograms 61
 and aided thresholds, 118
 as a predictor of performance, 269
 as predictors of speech detection, 118
Audiologic assessment, 77–84
Audition
 alternatives to, 4, 133–146
 of consonants, 163–167
 and speech reception, 2, 57, 157–167
 use of, 3
 of voice patterns, 159–161
 of vowels, 162–163
Auditory confusions, 99–100
Auditory discrimination
 of amplified speech, 83–84, 99–101, 157–167
 and reading, 257
 and speech production, 160
Auditory experience
 and auditory training, 112–113, 128–131
 and development of listening skills, 194–196, 210
 and reading, 245–261
 and speechreading, 137
 and use of residual hearing, 111–131
Auditory management, 114–115, 189–194
 see also Hearing aids
Auditory perception
 in infancy, 38
Auditory sensitivity, 57–60
 and pure tone tests, 60

communication, 26, 180–189,
198–199
evidence of comprehension, 185
sounds and hearing aid
selection, 104, 130–131
Normalization of speech, 175–178
Nursery class placement, 268, 281

O

Otologist
definition of, 77
examination of ear by, 64–65
Otoscope
use of, 64

P

Paraphrasing, 246
Parents, 9–11
acceptance of information, 12
and child's learning of language,
41–42
development of confidence, 12
and the development of reading
skills, 249, 256–257
and early communication,
12–13
education of, 272–275
and everyday interactions, 13
guidance of, 272–275
and hearing aids, 12
and importance of fathers, 211
involvement in diagnosis,
189–190
involvement throughout school
life, 11
language of, 230

and personnel involved with,
295
role in program selection, 266,
268
who are deaf, 189, 231–232
who are unavailable to child, 211
Part-time special class placement,
282–286
Personnel
preparation of specialist
teachers, 293–310
see also Support services
Phonemes
transcription of, 56
Phonetic level
evaluation of speech, 152–153
repertoire, 196–197, 202, 210
Phonic method of teaching
reading, 247–248, 261
Phonologic level assessment of
speech, 153–156, 213–214
Phonologic teaching strategies,
176–178, 213–214
Phonology, 33
transfer of phonetic level skills
to, 176–178, 213–214,
220–221
Phrases
early construction of, 47, 215
Physical status
as a variable in educational
placement, 269–270
Picture Lotto, 222–223
Place of consonant
production, 72
Plosives, 72
detection of, 116
Practice of motor speech skills,
141–143, 150–151
Pragmatic aspects of language,
232–233